The Radiologic Technologist's
Handbook of
SURGICAL PROCEDURES

Anthony C. Anderson, R.T. (R.), C.R.T.

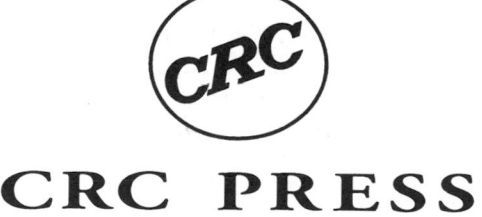

CRC PRESS

Boca Raton   London   New York   Washington, D.C.

Library of Congress Cataloging-in-Publication Data

Visit the CRC Press Web site at www.crcpress.com

No claim to original U.S. Government works
International Standard Book Number 0-8493-1506-9
Printed in the United States of America   5 6 7 8 9 0
Printed on acid-free paper

Introduction

This handbook was intended to be easily read and utilized as a quick reference. I have tried to organize and set down as concisely as possibly what I consider to be not only basic information, but also relevant details of surgical radiography. Whenever possible, this handbook suggests the best single position for performing specific surgical examinations. The illustrations were also selected to reflect this concept. Familiarization with patient positioning will ease the transition of the technologist from diagnostic imaging to surgical radiography.

To fully utilize the advancements in the ever-changing world of technology and their effects on the medical field and the practice of radiologic technology, it is important for the radiologic technologist to keep pace. During the past few years, the rapid development of sophisticated imaging modalities has made radiology the fastest-growing specialty in medicine.

The advancement of fluoroscopic imaging has greatly expanded the capabilities of relatively noninvasive diagnostic imaging within the surgical arena. New techniques in orthopedics, such as laparascopic spinal fusions, total joint replacements, and limb reattachments rely on the radiologic technologist's ability to fully utilize the fluoroscopic equipment. The general surgery field has also benefited from the technology of radiology in areas such as laparascopic cholangiogram, heart studies, and prostate sccd implantations. These examinations have become effective diagnostic and therapeutic alternatives to the extensive surgical procedures in selected patients. This handbook is designed as a guide to assist the technologist in meeting the challenges of this rapidly changing field.

This book can also serve as a general overview of the spectrum of imaging for a wide variety of surgical care providers. The surgeon will find it a useful guide in planning the proper imaging approach to specific surgical examinations. More than ever, surgeons are aware of the extensive role of diagnostic imaging modalities in their daily practices.

The advancements being made in X-ray technology make the importance of the radiologic technologist during surgery immeasurable. With these advancements, the level of skill and knowledge of the radiologic technologist has a great impact on the outcome of the surgical patient. It is understood that situations within the operating room change and cannot always be predicted, but, using this handbook as a foundation, radiologic technologists will be able to master many operating-room procedures.

Anthony C. Anderson

Author

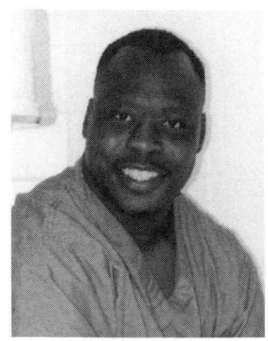

Anthony C. Anderson, C.R.T., R.T.(R.), is a certified and registered radiologic technologist with more than 10 years' experience performing surgical procedures.

Originally from Coolidge, Georgia, Anderson attended College of the Canyons in Valencia, California, then earned his BA degree in education at the University of Washington. He received his radiologic training at the Academy of Health Sciences at Fort Sam Houston, Texas, after joining the U.S. Army Reserves. Shortly after completing his training, Anderson was called to active duty for service in the Gulf War, where he performed surgical radiology at Riyadh Military Hospital in Saudi Arabia. On his return to the U.S., he went to work as a surgical radiologic technologist at Swedish Medical center in Seattle, a recognized leader in surgical innovations.

Currently, Anderson teaches a certified course on surgical technology for American Educators that trains radiologic technologists on techniques for using the c-arm and conducting intra-operative examinations. He is also the X-ray technologist for the Seattle Seahawks of the NFL. He continues to work at Swedish Medical Center and reside in the Seattle area with his wife, Tracy, and their daughter, Kayla.

Acknowledgments

I would like to thank the following groups of physicians: Northwest Spine & Pediatric Orthopaedics, Orthopaedic Physicians Associates, Seattle Orthopaedic and Fracture Clinic, Orthopaedic International, The Poly Clinic and Washington Orthopaedic. Doctors Howard Anderson, John Burns, Jim Crutcher, Mark Dales, Stewart Dupen, Daniel Flugstad, Scott Hormel, Howard King, Wally Krengel, Kenneth Leung, Marty Mankey, St. Elmo Newton, James Raisis, Hugh Toomey, Ted Wagner, William Wilson and Richard Zorn have all been very helpful.

A special thanks to Dr. Robert Winquist for his encouragement, and for being an enormous source of knowledge. Thank you, Cindy Morrell and Carmelita Byrd, and thanks to Ziehm International Medical Systems and Swedish Medical Center, Kayla Anderson, Willie Dean Glenn, and Minnie Roan. And last, but certainly not least, I would like to thank Tracy Van Horn for her support and hard work. Without them, this project would never have been completed.

Contents

PART I: Fluoroscopic Examinations

Part II: Intra-Operative Examinations

Part I:
Fluoroscopic Examinations

1. FEMORAL NAILING
(AP POSITION)

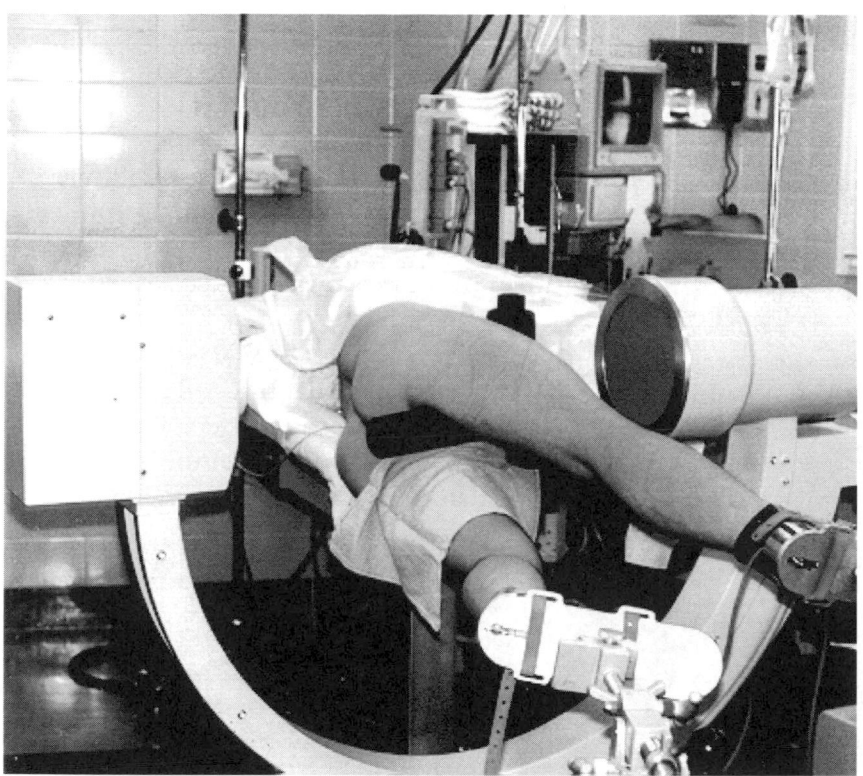

Figure 1.1 *C-arm in ap projection of hip.*

PATIENT POSITION:
Patient will be in lateral position with affected femur up and slightly forward.

C-ARM POSITION:
C-arm will enter facing patient. Rotate c-arm underneath the table to the ap projections. Ensure that c-arm is perpendicular to femur.

Notes: When moving from ap to lateral position, make sure not to bump instrumentation.

Position c-arm viewing cart at feet of patient with the doctor standing posterior to the patient.

Create distance and magnify image when creating round holes for distal locking screws.

During reaming, obtain true lateral of knee by tilting and rotating c-arm.

Position the c-arm to view reamers crossing fracture site.

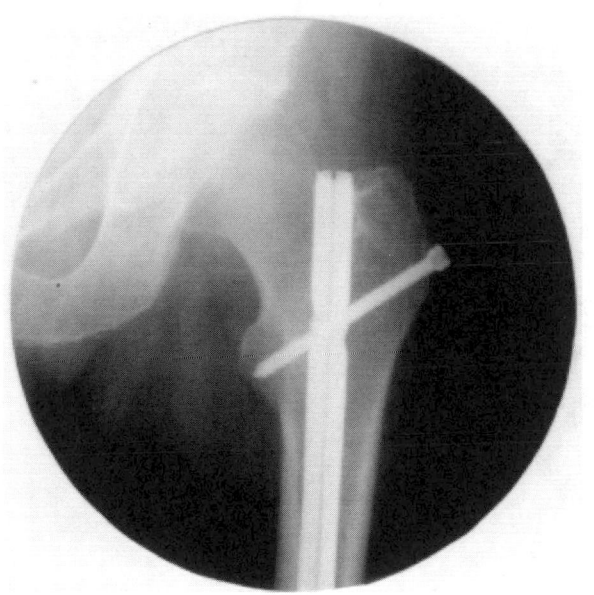

Figure 1.2 *C-arm image of ap hip with nail inserted.*

2. FEMORAL NAILING
(LATERAL POSITION)

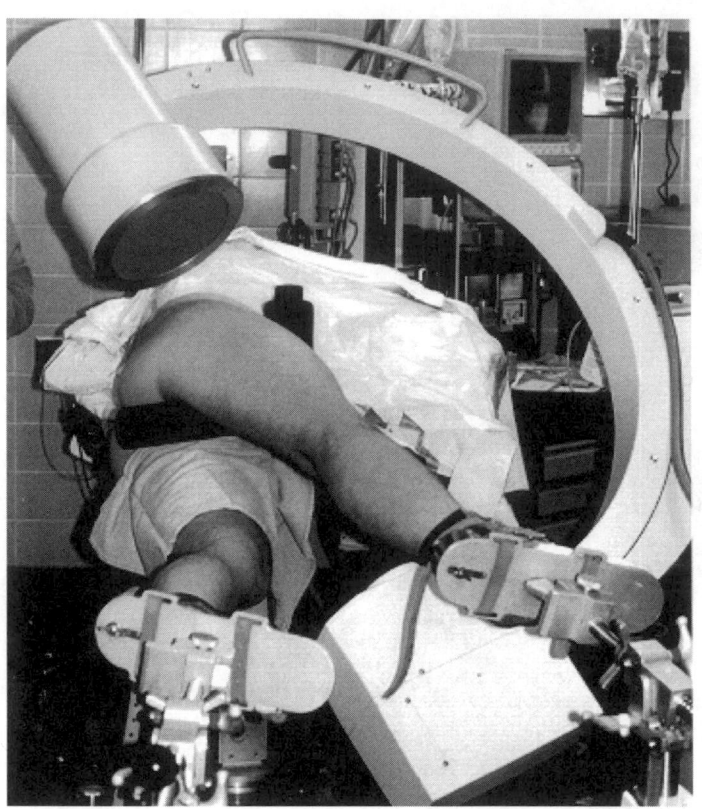

Figure 2.1 *C-arm in lateral projection with Winquist tilt view.*

PATIENT POSITION: Patient will be in lateral position with affected femur up and slightly forward.

C-ARM POSITION: C-arm will enter facing patient. Rotate c-arm 10 to 15 degrees over top of patient. Tilt c-arm 5 to 10 degrees toward head of femur.

This view, called the Winquist View, is used to throw the unaffected femur out of view, to elongate the femoral neck for true lateral viewing of starting position and to check anterior and posterior position.

Notes: When moving from ap to lateral position, make sure not to bump instrumentation.

Position c-arm viewing cart at feet of patient.

Doctor will stand posterior to patient.

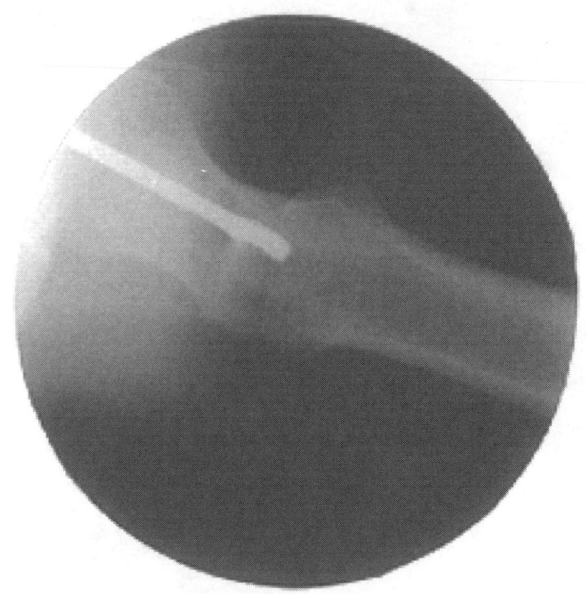

Figure 2.2 *C-arm image of lateral hip with starting auld in place.*

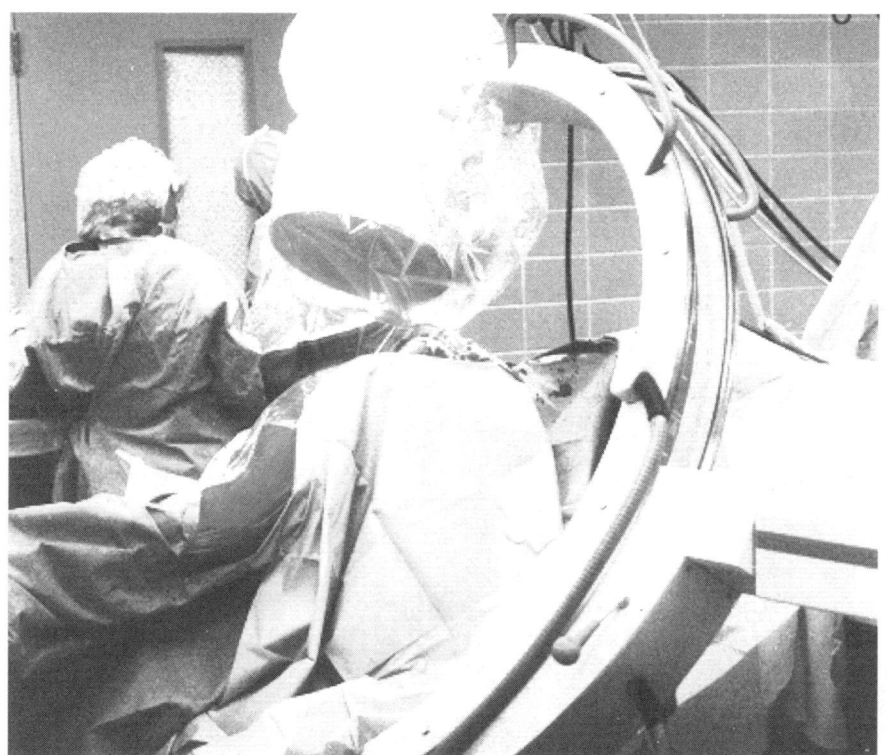

Figure 2.3 *The c-arm is in the Winquist view, which is best utilized to check anterior and posterior positions in relationship to the femoral shaft. The c-arm is rotated over the top and tilted to elongate the femur.*

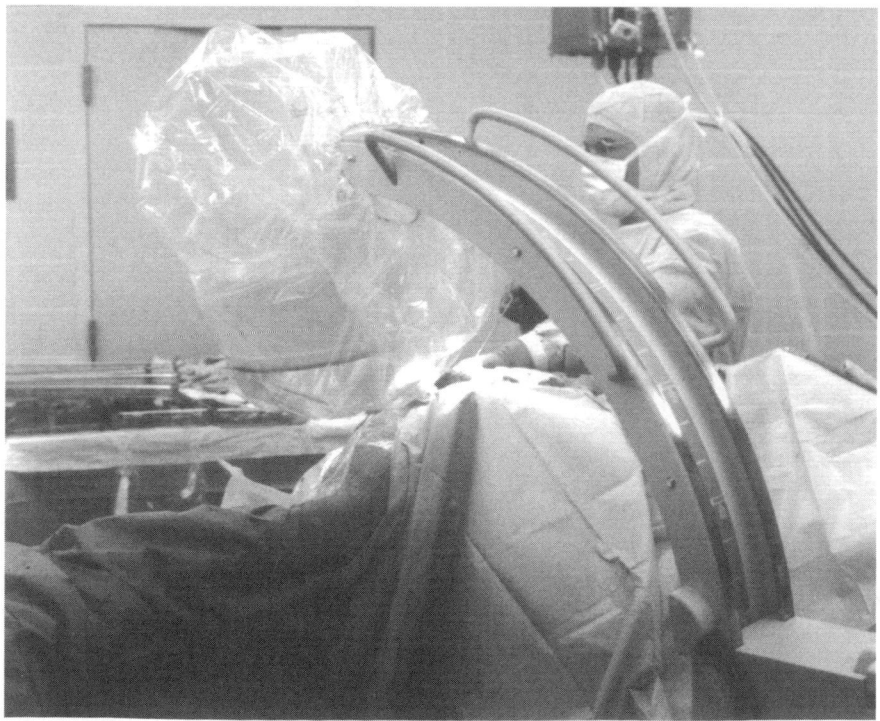

Figure 2.4 *The c-arm in a true lateral view in relationship to femur position. The c-arm is tilted to align with the femur. This will give a better indication of fracture alignment and reamer size.*

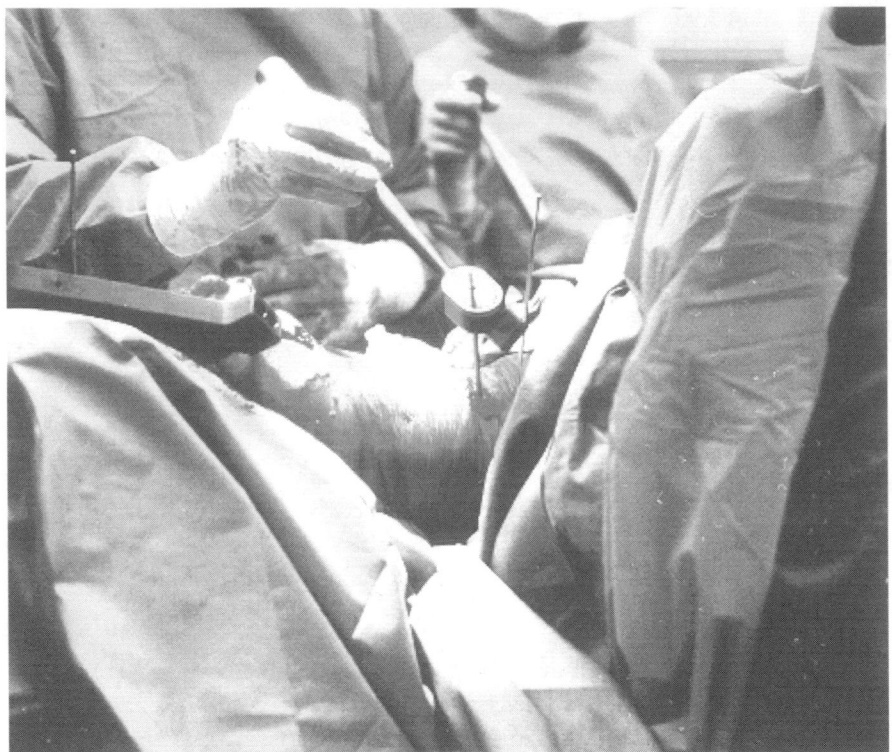

Figure 2.5. *During distal targeting for femoral nail, raise the c-arm away from the knee to enlarge the hole and create working space. Use the magnify button on the c-arm if available.*

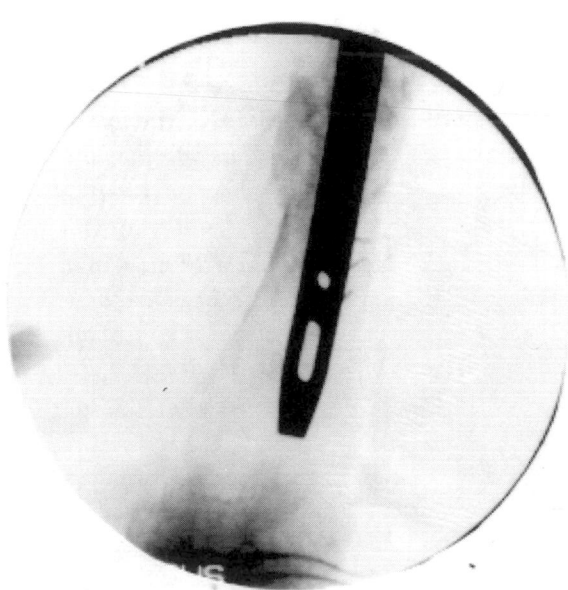

Figure 2.6 *Incorrect hole alignment. Note how hole is oblong.*

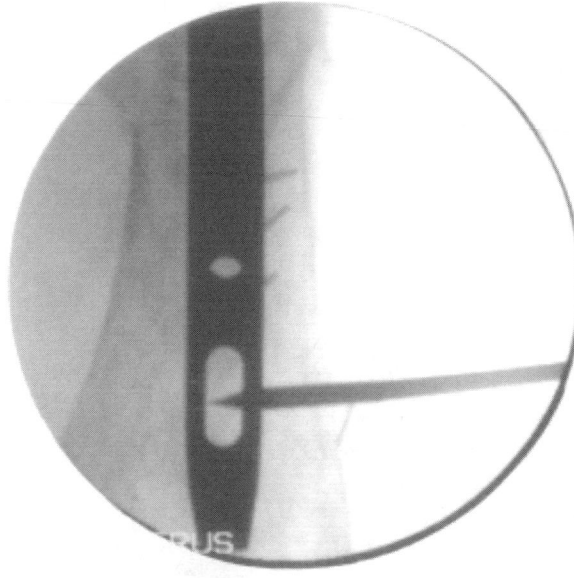

Figure 2.7 *Correct hole alignment. Note that hole is now rounded.*

3. SUPRACONDYLAR FEMORAL NAIL
(AP VIEW)

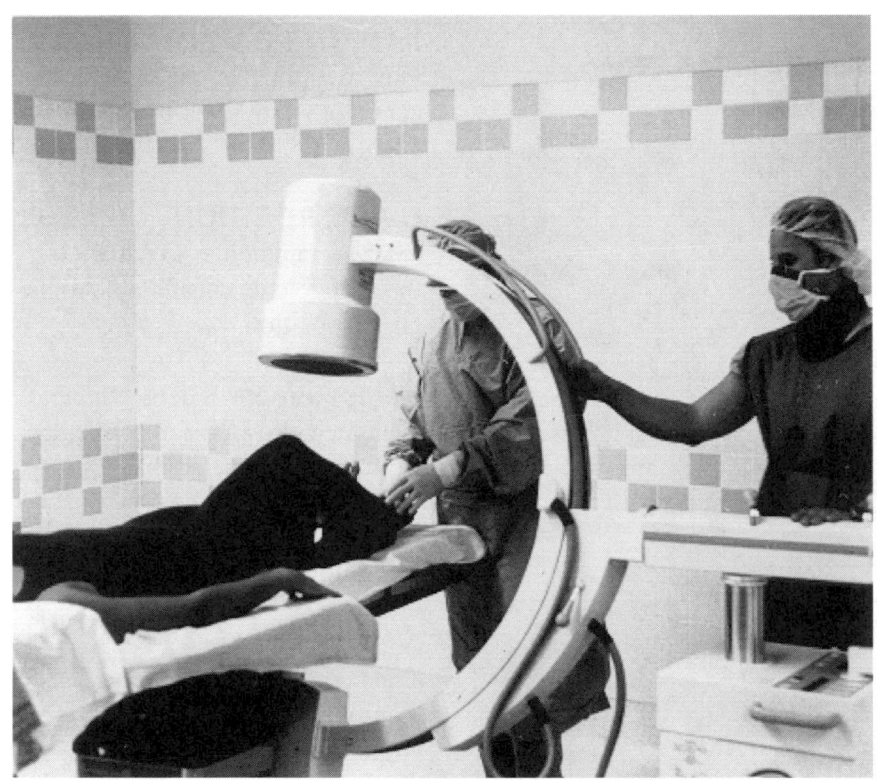

Figure 3.1 *C-arm in ap projection of distal femur.*

PATIENT POSITION: Patient will be supine with the affected knee slightly bent on radiolucent table.

C-ARM POSITION: C-arm will enter perpendicular to patient and in the ap position.

Notes: Ensure underneath clearance allows for movement from the knee to the hip.

C-arm may have to be rotated over or backward to create a true ap view.

Tilt c-arm to open joint space of knee for starting point.

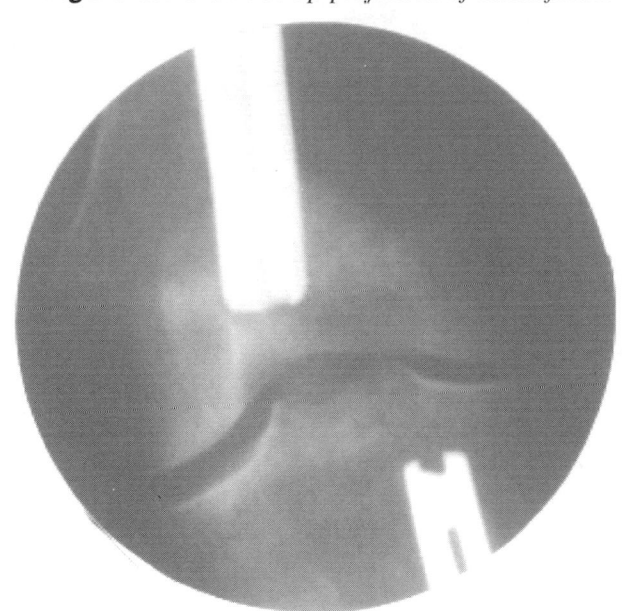

Figure 3.2 *X-ray image of distal femur.*

4. SUPRACONDYLAR FEMORAL NAIL
(LATERAL VIEW)

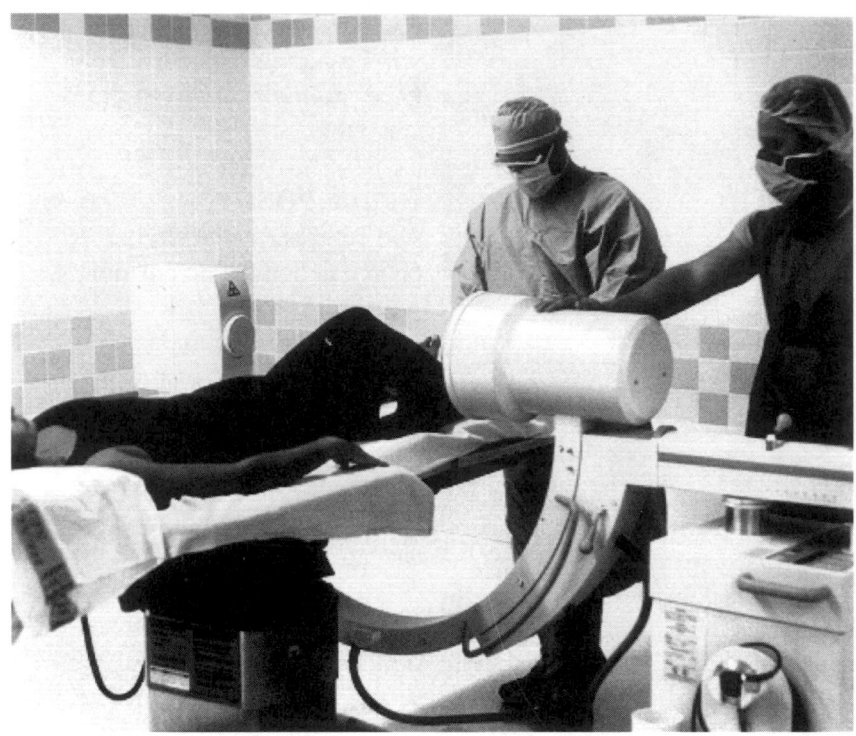

Figure 4.1 *C-arm in lateral projection of distal femur.*

PATIENT POSITION:
Patient will be supine on radiolucent table with the affected knee slightly bent.

C-ARM POSITION: C-arm will enter perpendicular to patient, then rotate underneath table to the lateral position.

Notes: Ensure underneath table clearance allows for movement from the knee to the hip.

Be careful not to bump instrumentation when moving from ap to lateral.

C-arm or knee may have to be manipulated to create a true lateral view.

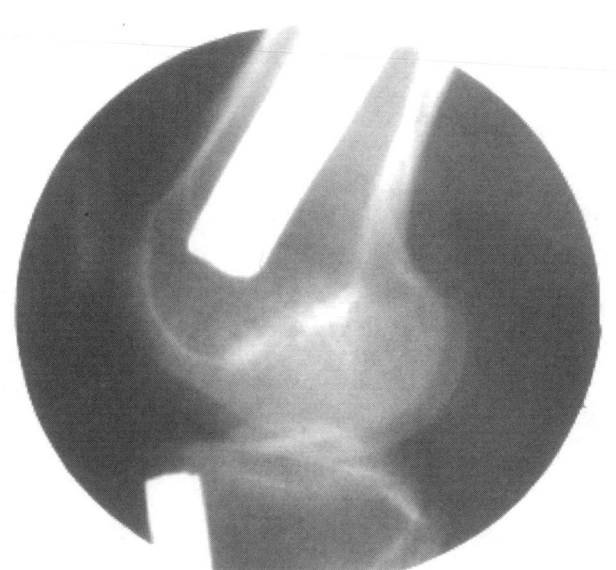

Figure 4.2 *X-ray image of distal femur.*

5. FEMORAL NAIL REMOVAL

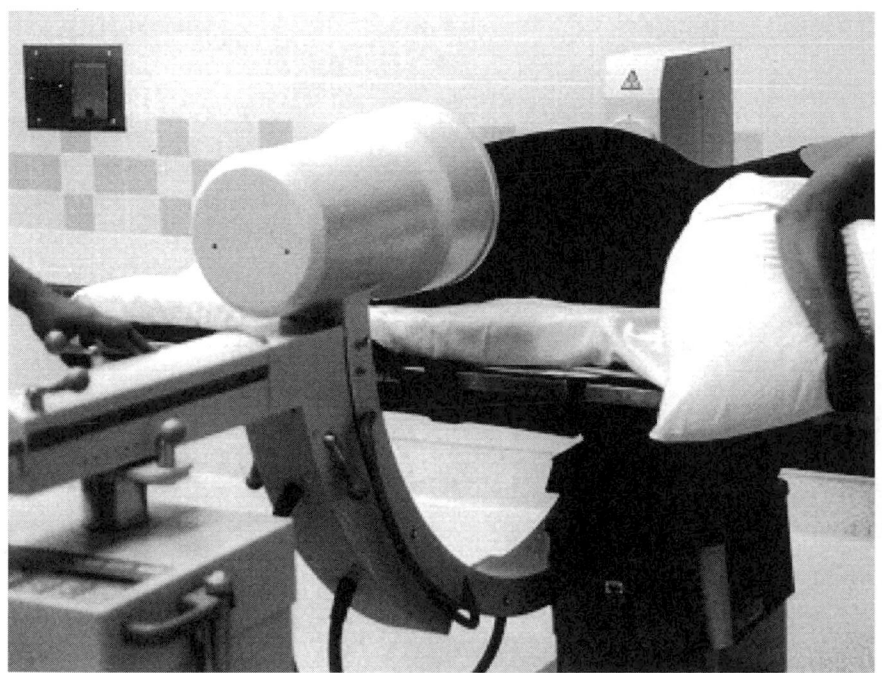

Figure 5.1 *C-arm in ap projection of femur.*

PATIENT POSITION:
Patient will be in lateral position with affected femur up.

C-ARM POSITION: C-arm should be positioned perpendicular to patient with patient facing c-arm.

Notes: Rotate c-arm 90 degrees to obtain ap view.

It may be necessary to tilt c-arm to obtain view of femoral head.

If table does not allow underneath movement, an over-the-top position can be utilized with manipulation of c-arm.

Tilting of the c-arm may be necessary to view head of femur in ap position.

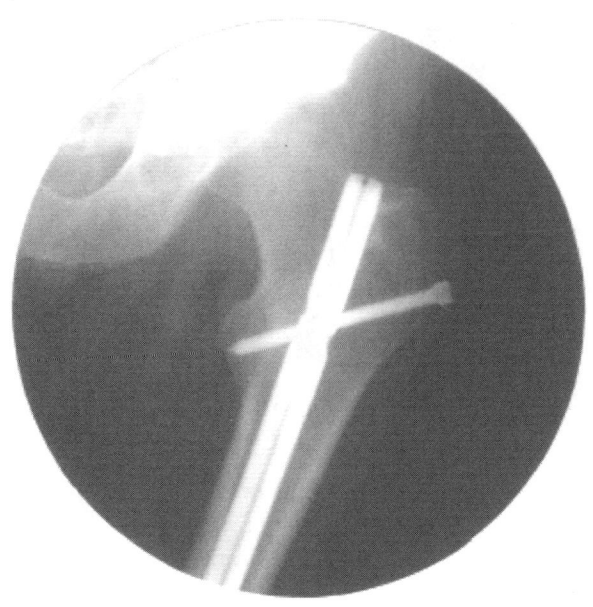

Figure 5.2 *C-arm image of ap hip with nail inserted.*

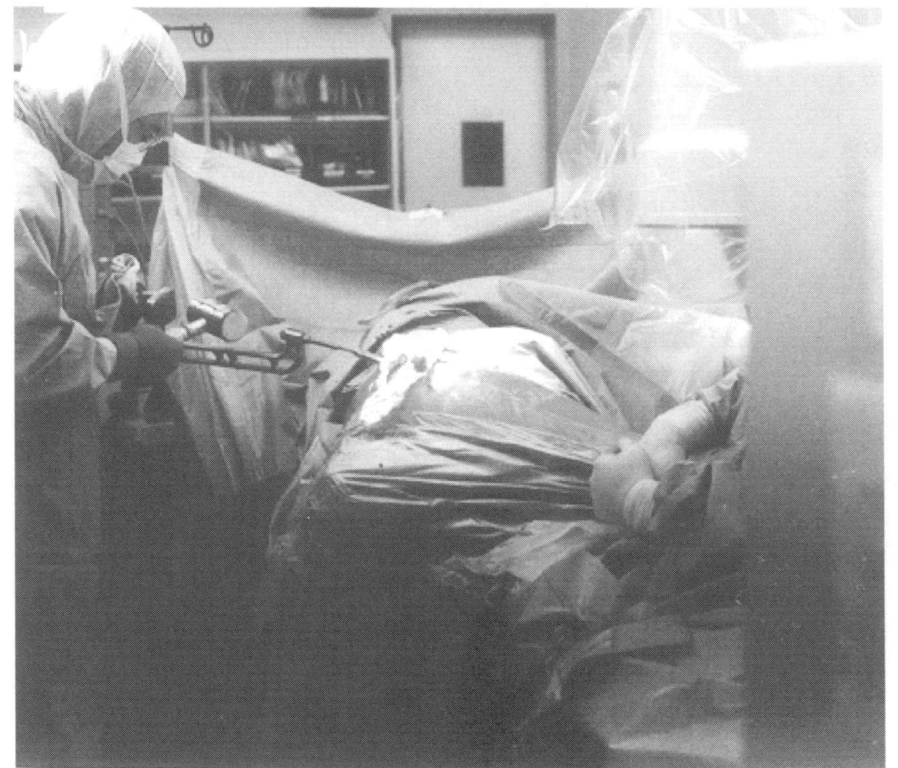

Figure 5.3 *The femoral nail being extracted from the femur.*

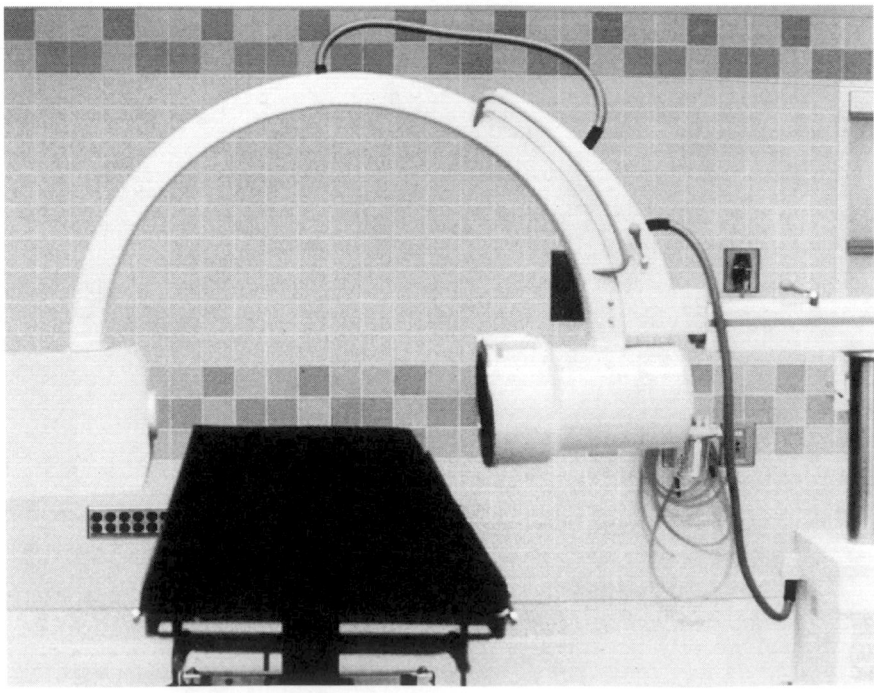

Figure 5.4 *Note that if the table does not allow for underneath movement, the over-the-top position may have to be utilized.*

6. TIBIAL NAILING
(AP POSITION)

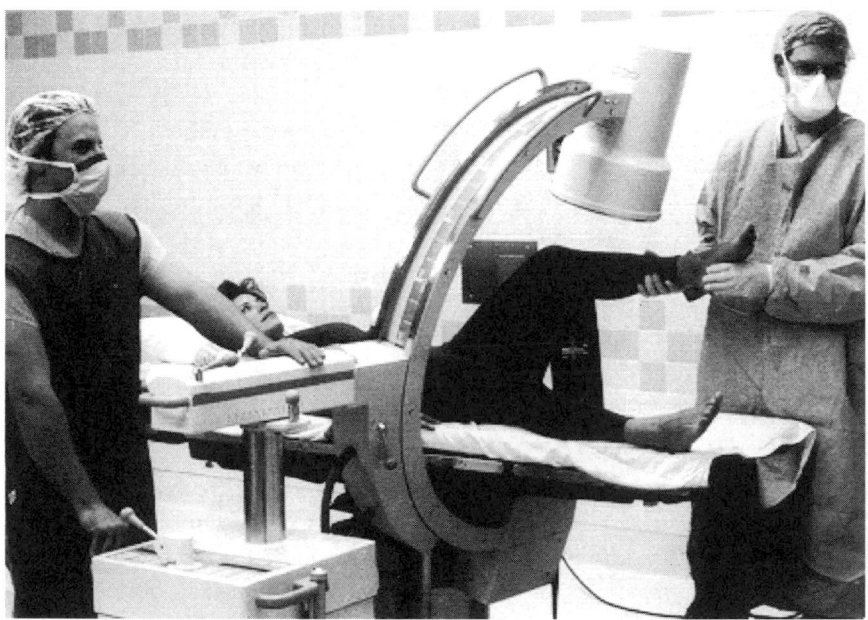

Figure 6.1 *C-arm in ap projection of tibia.*

PATIENT POSITION: Patient will be supine with affected leg flexed at the knee.

C-ARM POSITION: C-arm will enter perpendicular to patient on opposite side of physician.

Notes: During ap view, tilt c-arm to the angle of the tibia to obtain true perspective.

Rotate c-arm 90 degrees to obtain lateral view.

When moving from ap to lateral view make sure not to distract instrumentation.

While obtaining round holes for locking screws, increase distance, then magnify image.

Rotation of the leg along with manipulation of c-arm may be required to obtain perfect round holes.

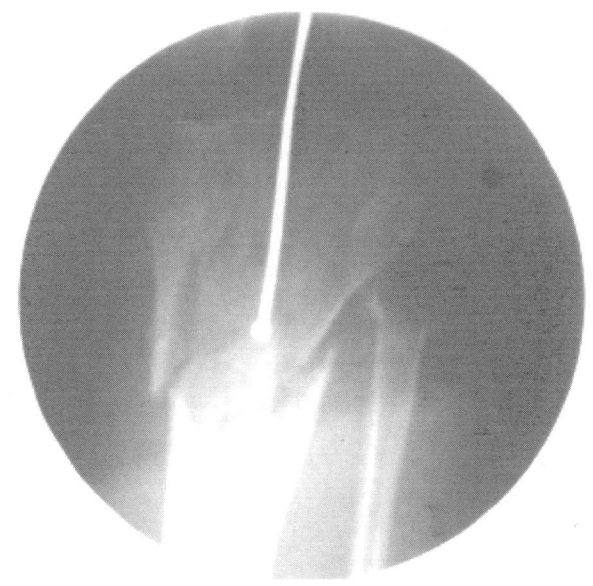

Figure 6.2 *C-arm image of tibia with bulb tip inserted.*

7. TIBIAL NAILING
(LATERAL POSITION)

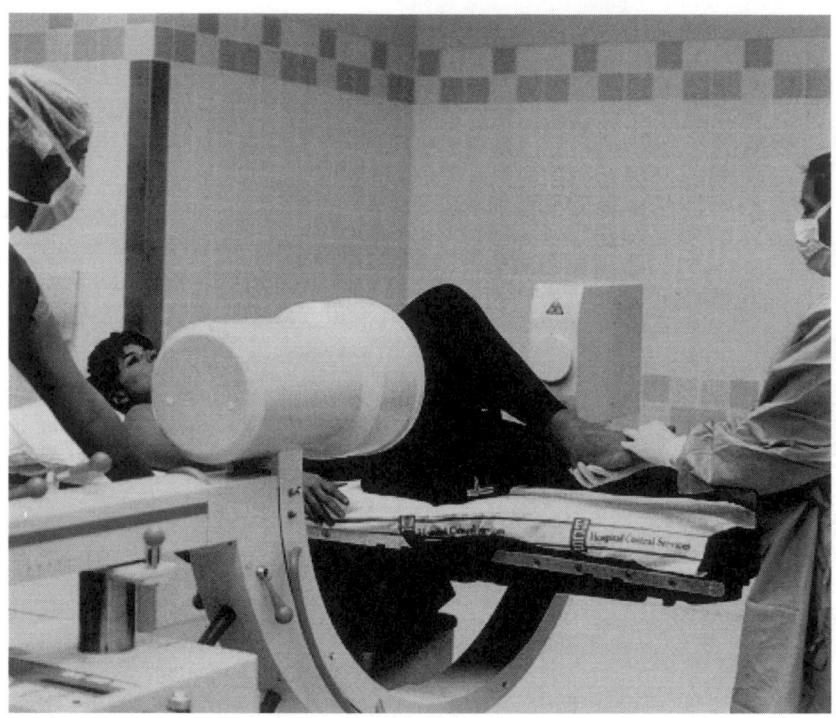

Figure 7.1 *C-arm in lateral projection of tibia.*

PATIENT POSITION: Patient will be supine with affected leg flexed at the knee.

C-ARM POSITION: C-arm will enter in ap projection then rotate underneath table for lateral view.

Notes: Ensure area underneath table is clear to allow movement.

It may be necessary to angle c-arm to create true lateral view.

When moving from ap to lateral view make sure not to distract instrumentation.

Place image intensifier close to knee to create a larger field of view.

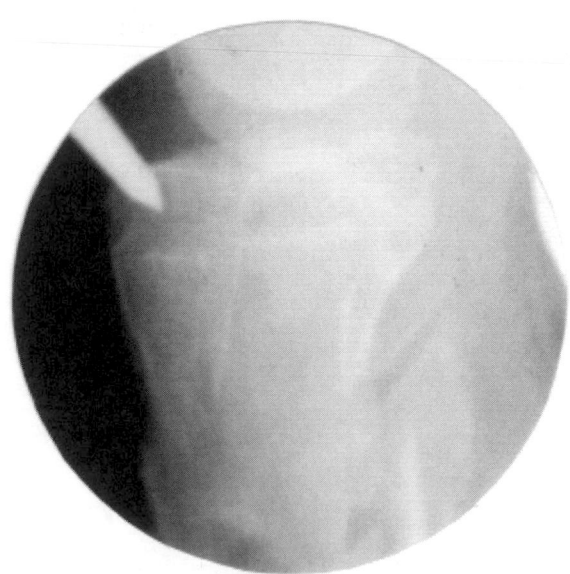

Figure 7.2 *C-arm image of lateral tibia with starting auld in place.*

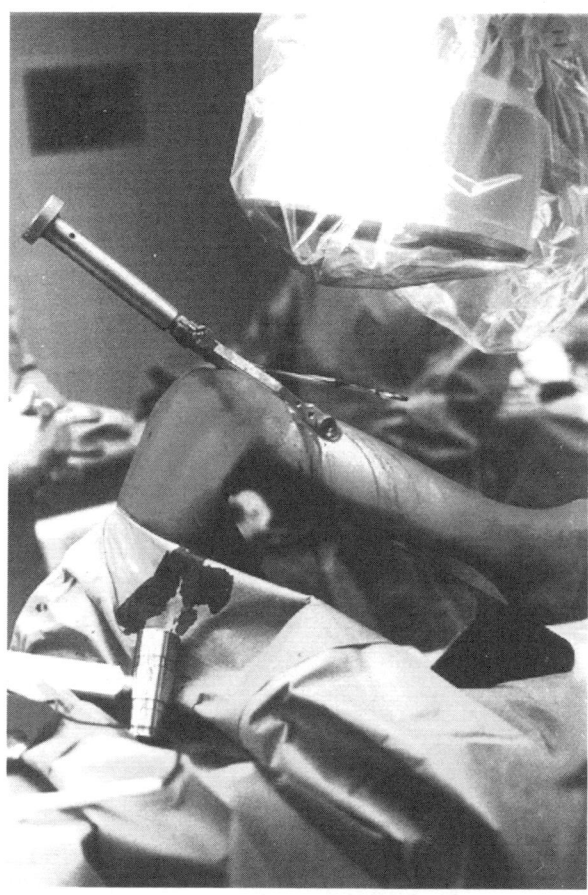

Figure 7.3 *The c-arm is tilted to align for a true ap of the tibia. Nail driver is in place for proximal targeting.*

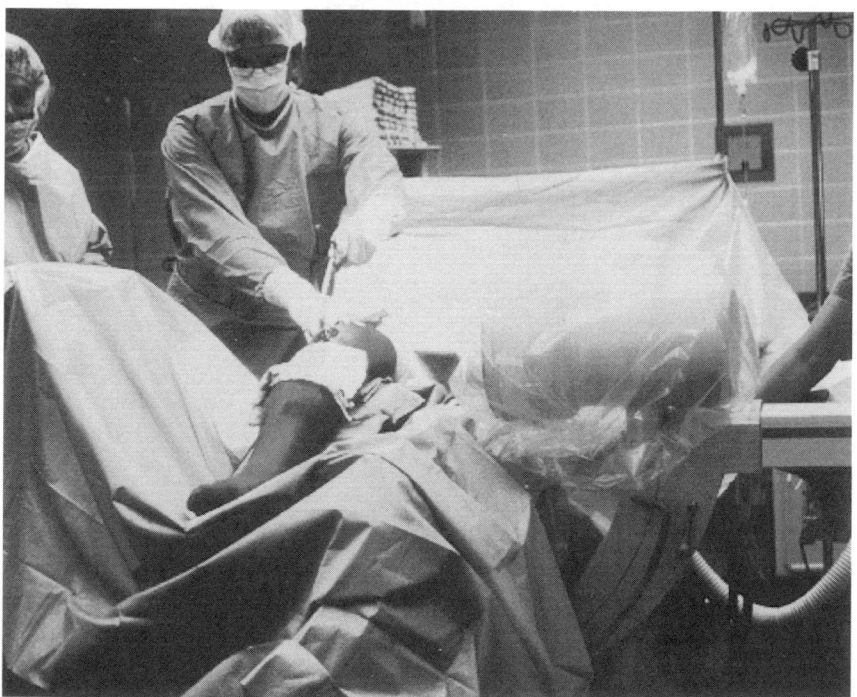

Figure 7.4
C-arm in position for lateral view of the tibia. Starting auld is being utilized.

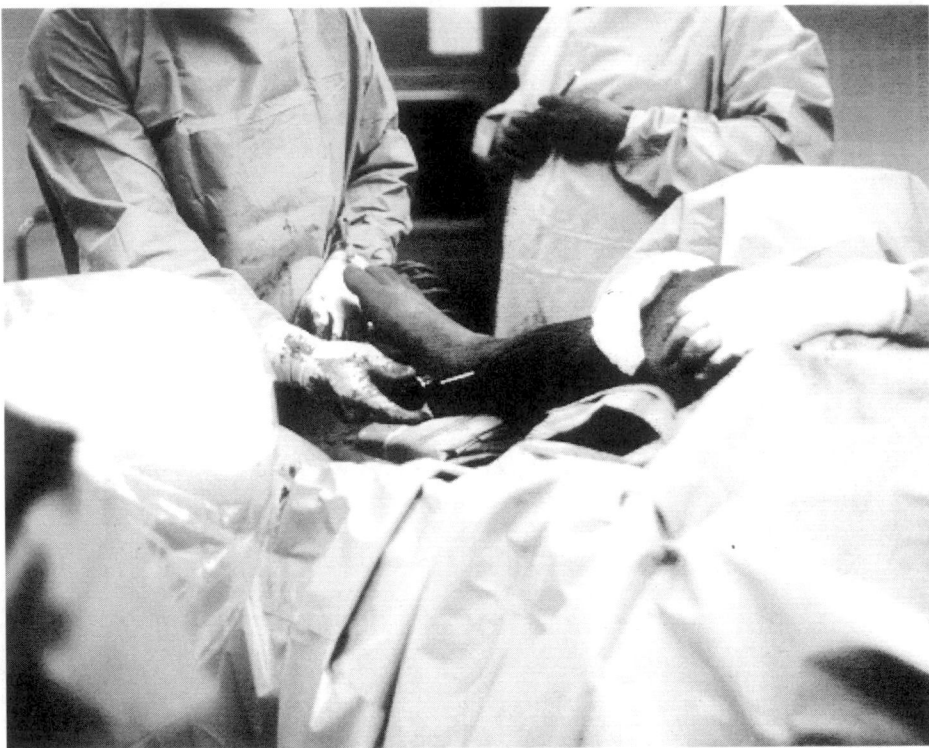

Figure 7.5 *During distal targeting for tibial nail, move image intensifier farthest from the ankle. This will enlarge the image for better targeting and create working space. Use magnification button on c-arm if available.*

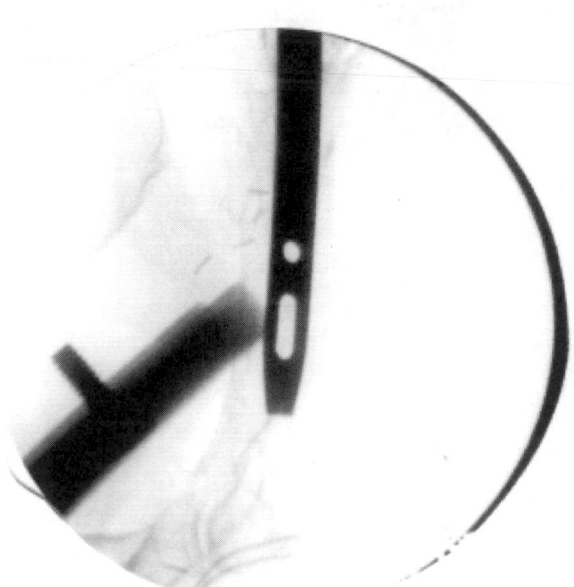

Figure 7.6 *Incorrect hole alignment. Note how hole is oblique.*

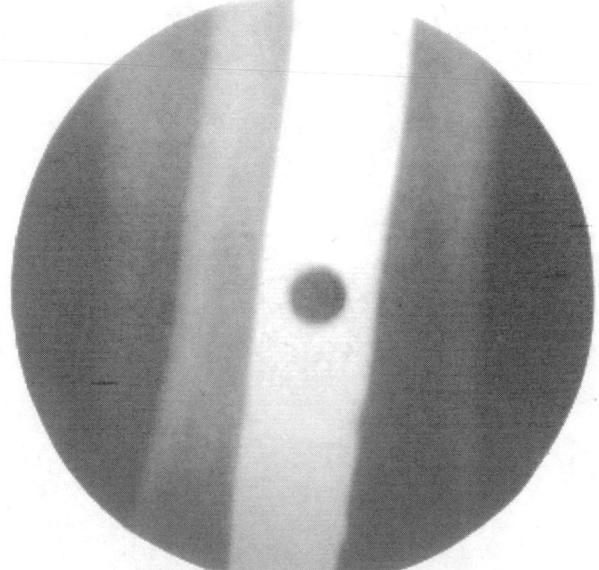

Figure 7.7 *Correct hole alignment. Note hole is perfectly round.*

8. HUMERAL NAILING

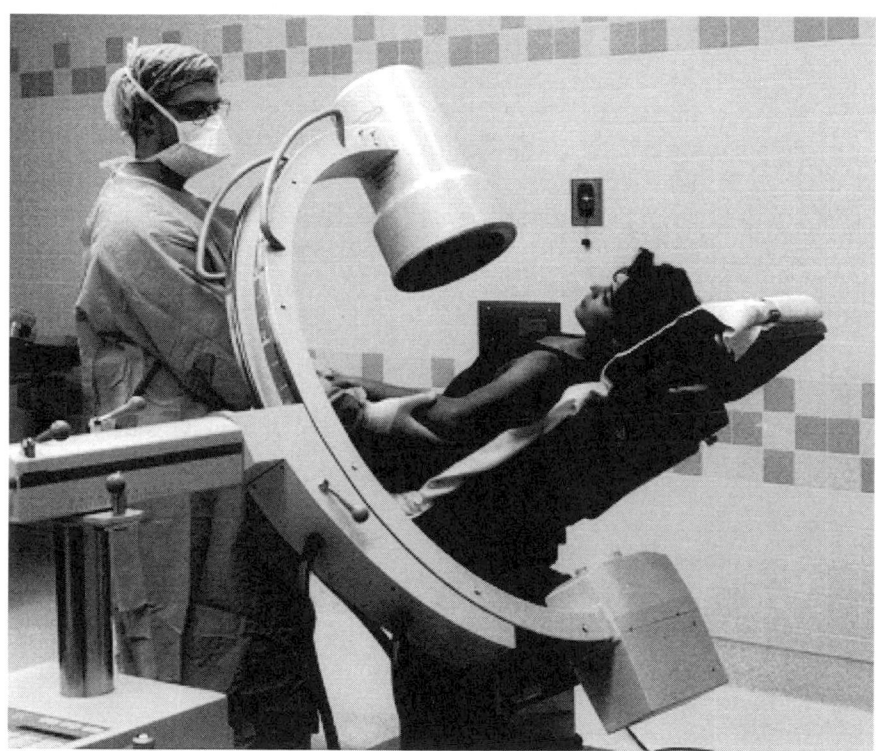

Figure 8.1 *C-arm in ap projection of humerus.*

PATIENT POSITION: Patient will be supine or in a semi-sitting position.

C-ARM POSITION: C-arm will enter on side of affected humerus either at a position perpendicular to, or at 45 degrees to patient.

Notes: To obtain true ap of humerus, it may be necessary to tilt c-arm slightly, depending on patient position.

Lateral view may be obtained by surgeon's rotation of humerus.

Magnify image of distal locking screws for better visualization.

When viewing humeral head, be aware of patient position, to avoid bumping patient's head.

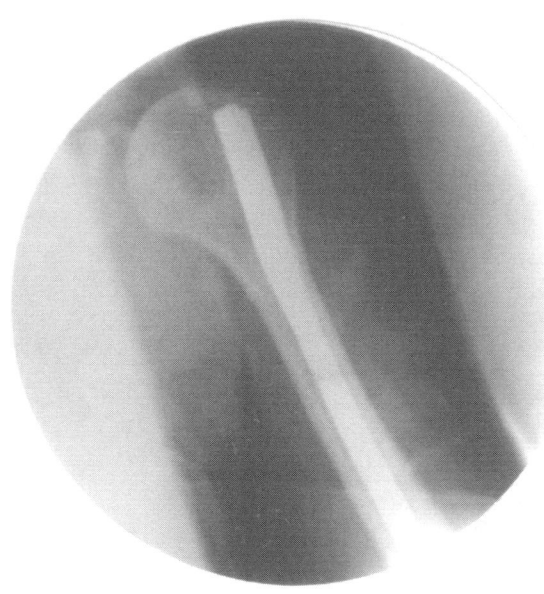

Figure 8.2 *C-arm image of humerus with nail in place.*

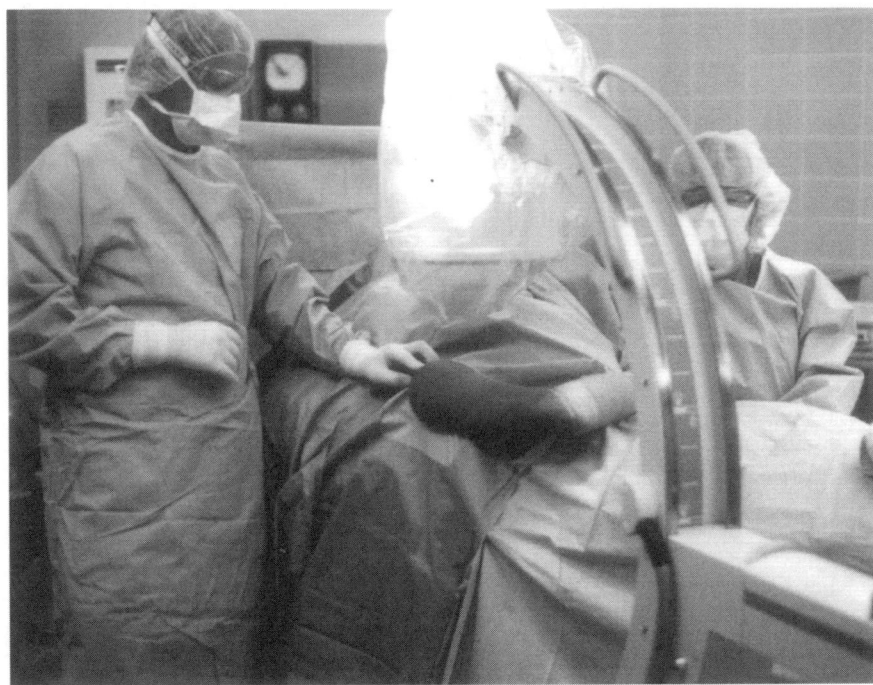

Figure 8.3 *Demonstrating how the lateral view is obtained during the humeral nail procedure. The assistant will rotate the arm across the body, bringing the elbow out.*

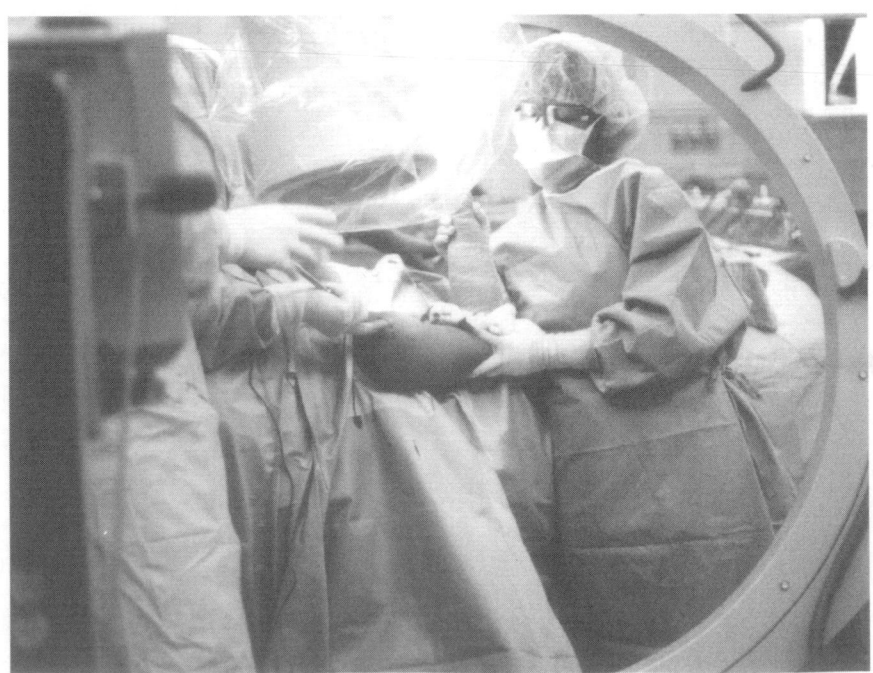

Figure 8.4 *To obtain the ap view of the humerus, the assistant will rotate the hand up. This brings the elbow along the body and shows the ap.*

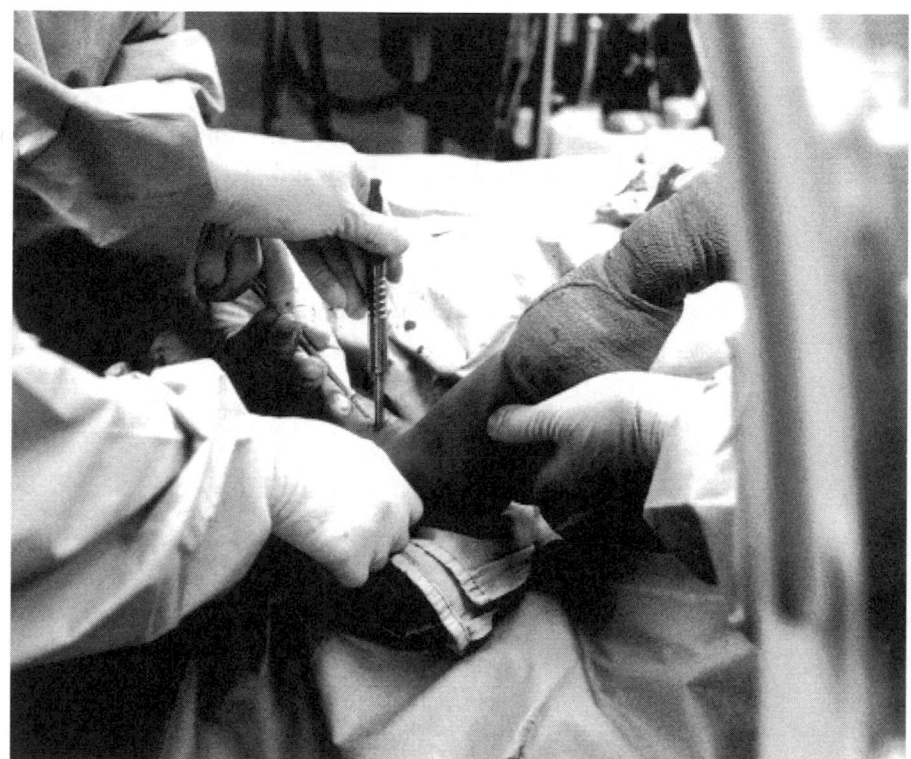

Figure 8.5 *During distal targeting for the humerus, raise the c-arm to move image intensifier farther from the humerus. This will enlarge the hole and create working space.*

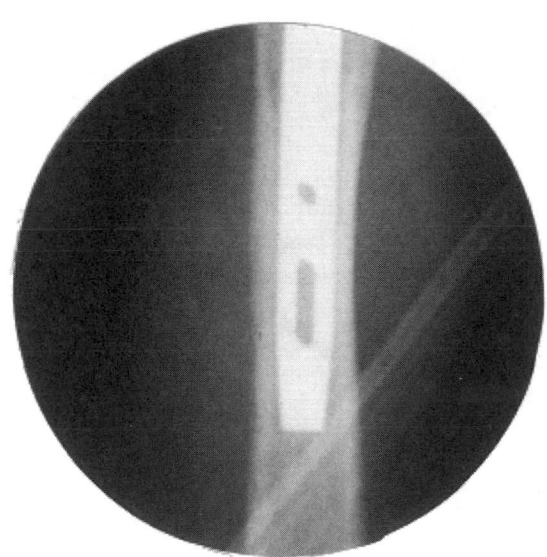

Figure 8.6 *Incorrect hole alignment Note how hole is oblique.*

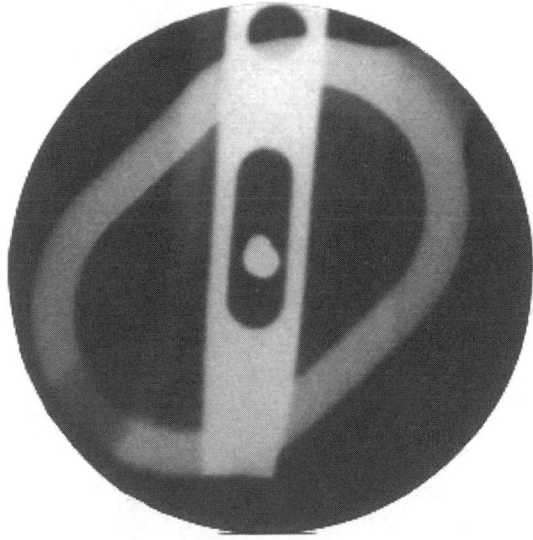

Figure 8.7 *Correct hole alignment. Note hole is now round.*

9. DECOMPRESSION HIP SCREW
(AP POSITION)

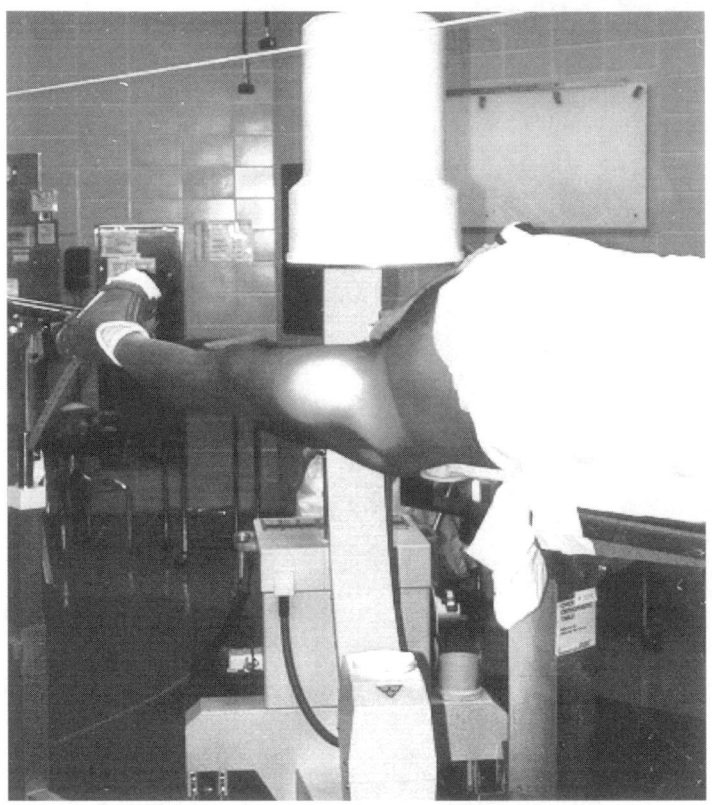

Figure 9.1 *C-arm in ap projection of hip.*

PATIENT POSITION:
Patient is supine with unaffected leg abducted to maximum tolerance.

C-ARM POSITION: Position c-arm parallel to unaffected hip with image intensifier positioned over affected hip.

Notes: Maximum abduction is critical to obtaining quality views.

Ensure that arm on side of affected hip is secured out of view.

Drape c-arm with snap cover drapes to allow ease of movement from ap to lateral view.

When moving from ap to lateral view, be sure not to bump instrumentation.

To obtain lateral view, rotate c-arm 90 degrees to lateral position.

Ensure area underneath table is clear to allow movement of c-arm.

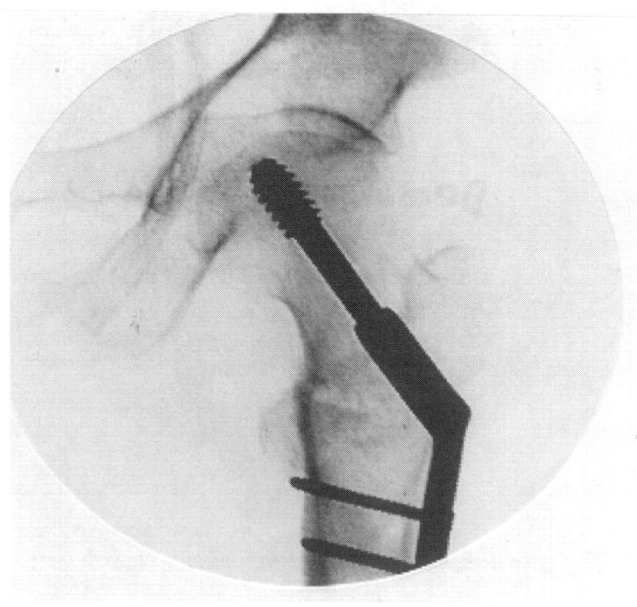

Figure 9.2 *X-ray image of ap hip with screw inserted.*

10. DECOMPRESSION HIP SCREW
(LATERAL POSITION)

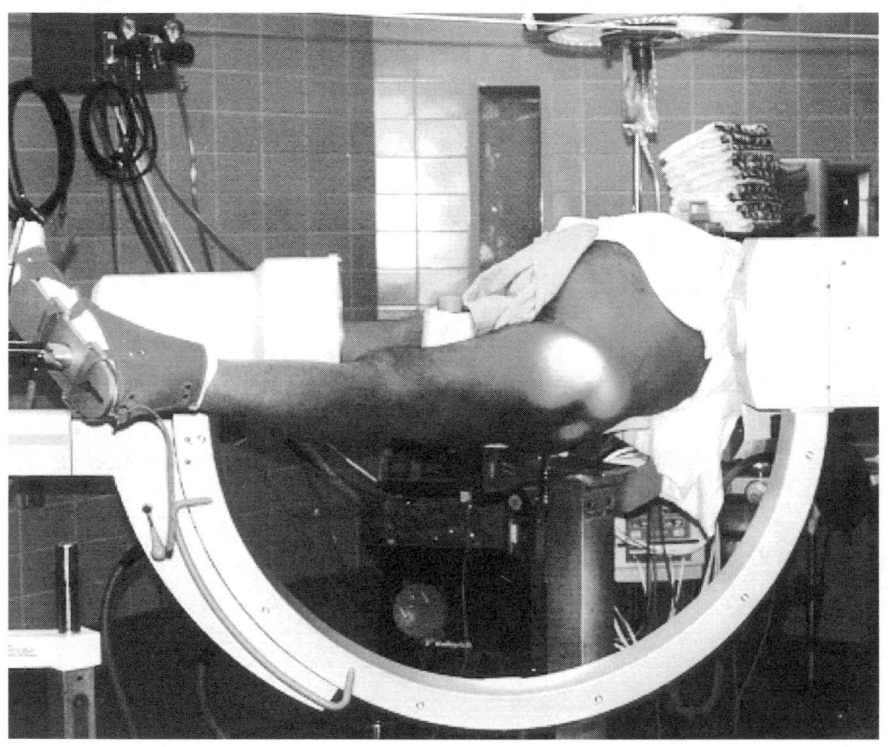

Figure 10.1 *C-arm in lateral projection of hip.*

PATIENT POSITION:
Patient will be supine with unaffected hip abducted to maximum tolerance.

C-ARM POSITION:
Position c-arm parallel to unaffected hip with "C" rotated underneath to lateral view.

Notes: Maximum abduction is critical to obtaining quality views.

Ensure that arm on side of affected hip is secured out of view.

Drape c-arm with snap-cover drapes to allow ease of movement from ap to lateral view.

It may be necessary to tilt c-arm inward to clearly see the femoral head in the lateral position.

When moving from ap to lateral view, take care not to bump instrumentation.

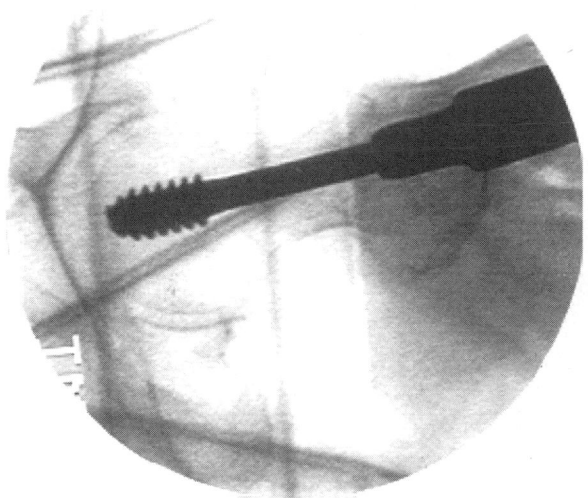

Figure 10.2 *X-ray image of lateral hip with screw inserted.*

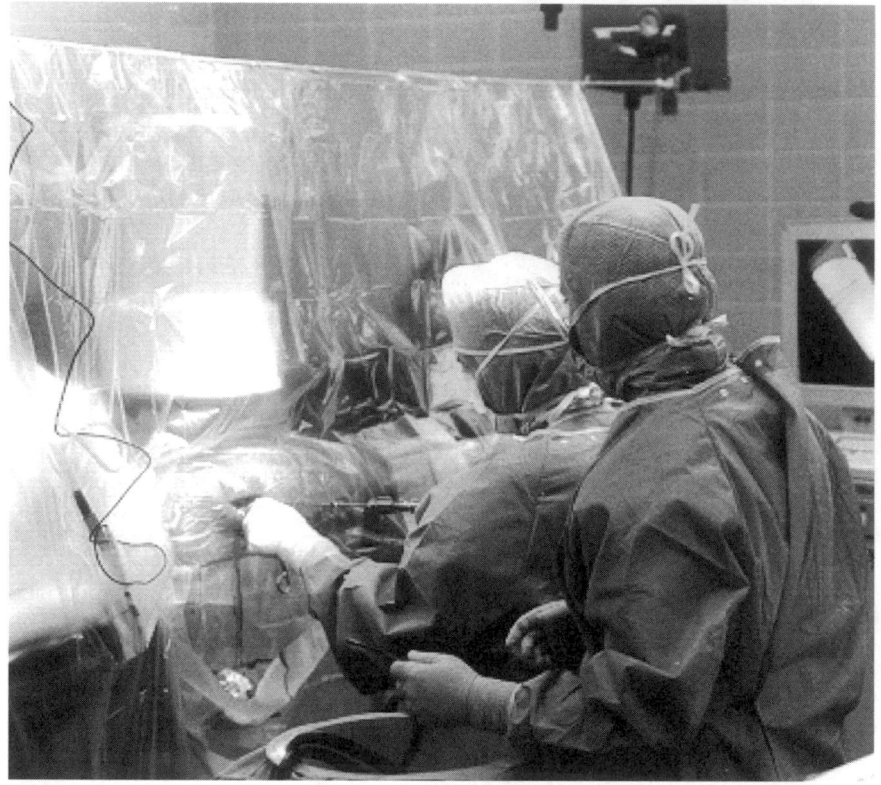

Figure 10.3 *When performing hip procedures using a vertical isolation drape, ensure drape allows for moving the image intensifier over the outer cortex.*

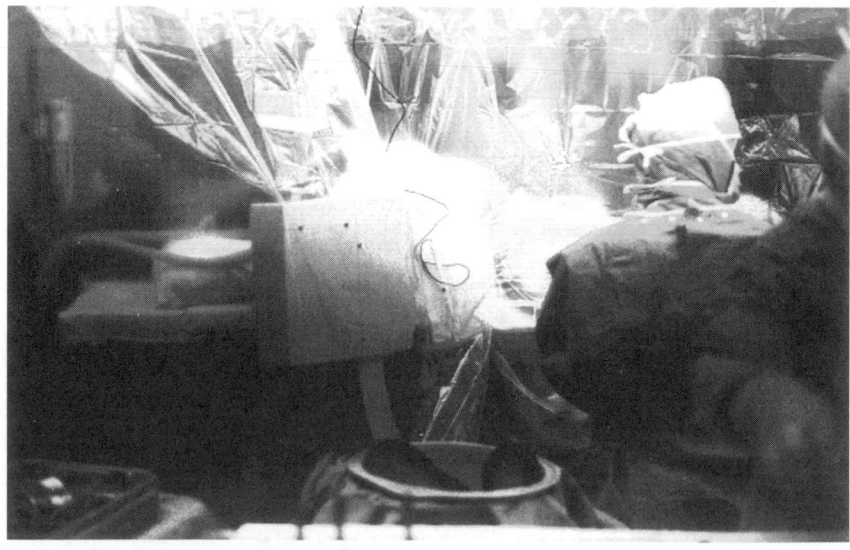

Figure 10.4 *The cautery instrumentation is interfering with lateral image. Ensure that area is clear during draping.*

11. CANNULATED HIP SCREWS
(AP POSITION)

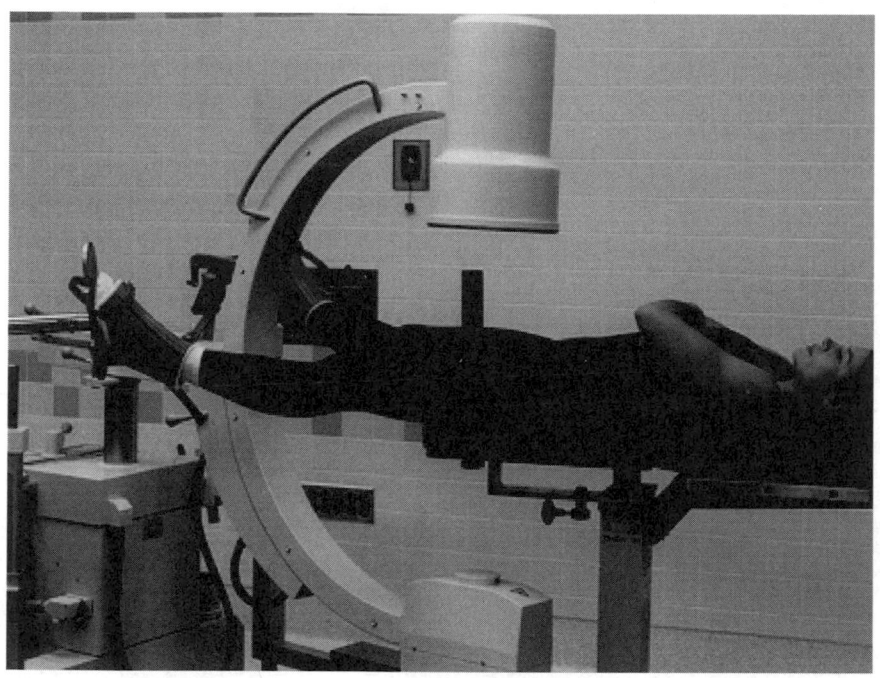

Figure 11.1 *C-arm in ap projection of hip.*

PATIENT POSITION: Patient is supine with unaffected leg abducted to maximum tolerance.

C-ARM POSITION: Position c-arm parallel to unaffected hip with image intensifier positioned over affected hip.

Notes: Maximum abduction of unaffected leg is critical to obtaining quality views.

Ensure that arm on side of affected hip is secured out of view.

Drape c-arm with snap cover drapes to allow ease of movement from ap to lateral view.

When moving from ap to lateral view, ensure not to bump instrumentation.

To obtain lateral view, rotate c-arm 90 degrees to lateral position.

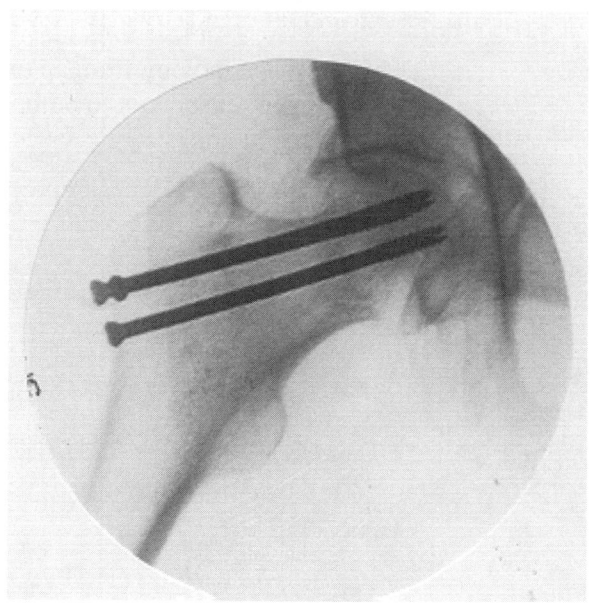

Figure 11.2 *C-arm image of ap hip with screws inserted.*

12. CANNULATED HIP SCREWS
(LATERAL POSITION)

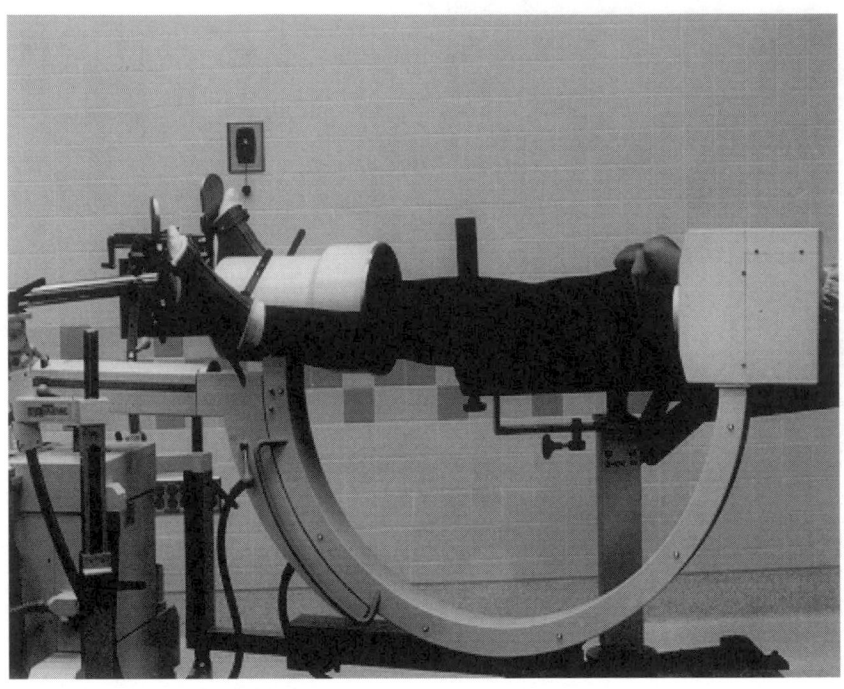

Figure 12.1 *C-arm in lateral projection of hip.*

PATIENT POSITION: Patient will be supine with unaffected leg abducted to maximum tolerance.

C-ARM POSITION: Position c-arm parallel to unaffected leg with "C" rotated underneath table to lateral position.

Notes: Maximum abduction is critical to obtaining quality views.

Ensure that arm on side of affected hip is secured out of view.

Drape c-arm with snap-cover drapes to allow ease of movement from ap to lateral view.

It may be necessary to tilt c-arm in to clearly see the femoral head in the lateral position.

When moving from ap to lateral view, ensure not to bump instrumentation.

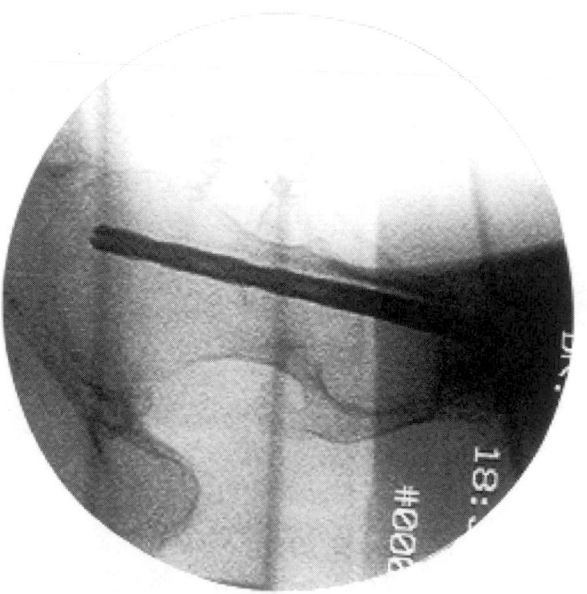

Figure 12.2 *X-ray image of lateral hip with screws inserted.*

13. HIP PINNING
(AP POSITION)

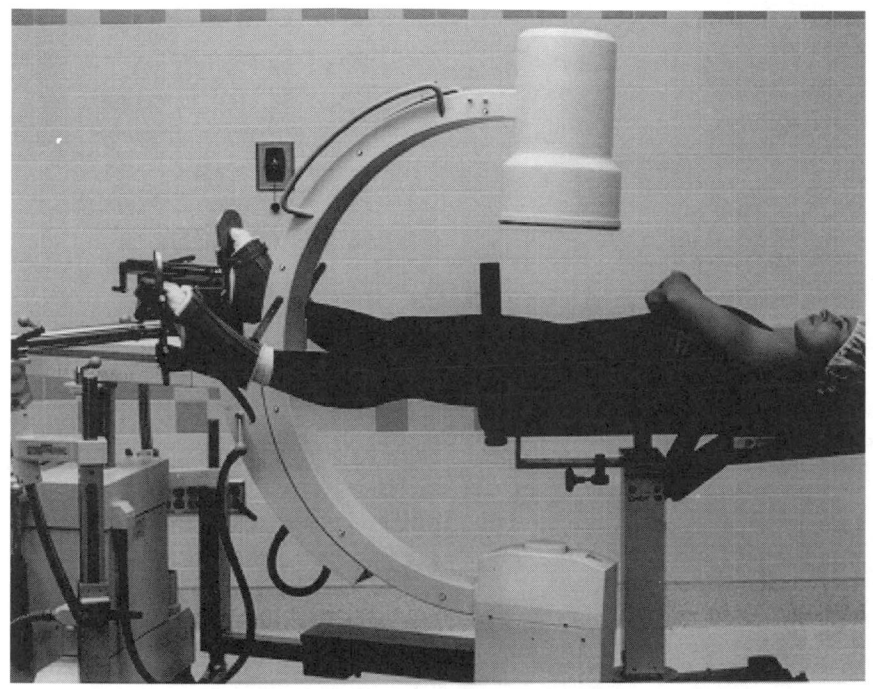

Figure 13.1 *C-arm in ap projection of hip.*

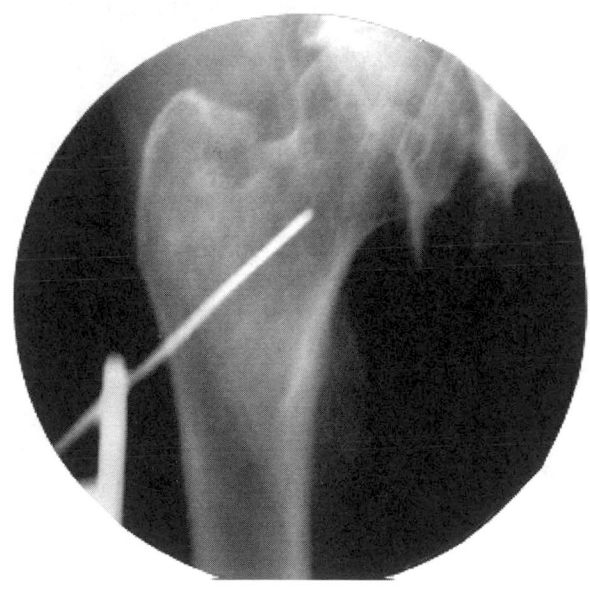

Figure 13.2 *C-arm image of ap hip with pin in place.*

PATIENT POSITION: Patient is supine with legs abducted to maximum tolerance.

C-ARM POSITION: Position c-arm parallel to unaffected hip with image intensifier positioned over affected hip.

Notes: Maximum abduction is critical to obtaining quality views.

Ensure that arm on side of affected hip is secured out view.

Drape c-arm with snap cover drapes to allow ease of movement from ap to lateral view.

When moving from ap to lateral view make sure not to bump instrumentation.

To obtain lateral view rotate c-arm 90 degrees to lateral position.

14. HIP PINNING
(LATERAL POSITION)

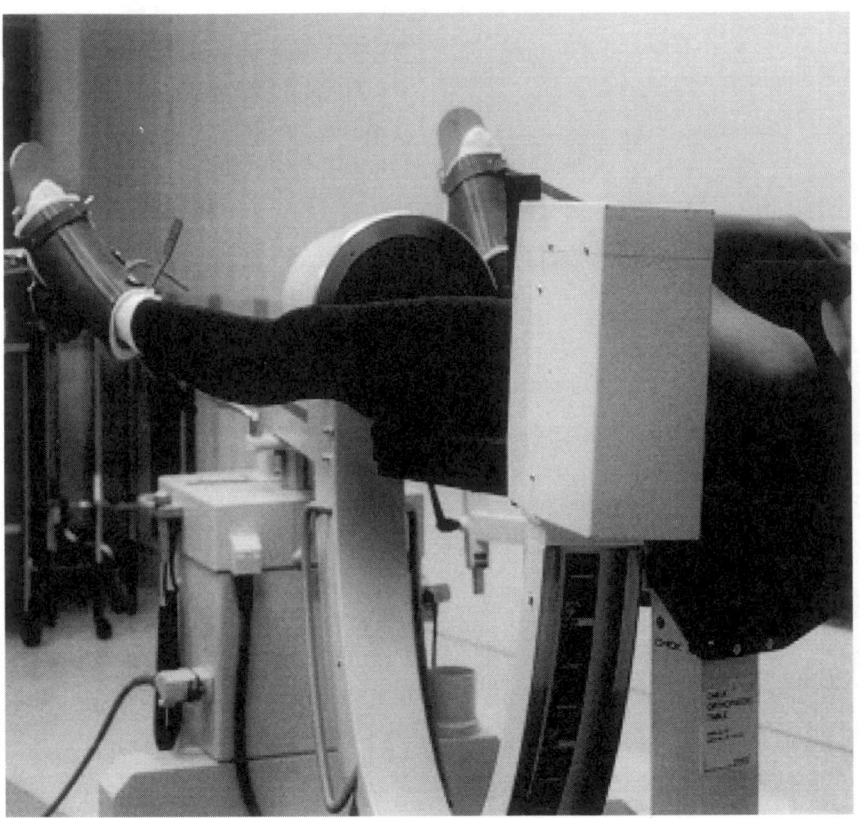

Figure 14.1 *C-arm in lateral projection of hip.*

PATIENT POSITION: Patient will be supine with legs abducted.

C-ARM POSITION: Position c-arm parallel to unaffected hip. Move image intensifier closer to hip for larger field of view.

Notes: Maximum abduction is critical to obtaining quality views.

Ensure that arm on side of affected hip is secured out of view.

Drape c-arm with snap cover drapes to allow ease of movement from ap to lateral view.

It may be necessary to tilt c-arm in to clearly see the femoral head in the lateral position.

When moving from ap to lateral view make sure not to bump instrumentation.

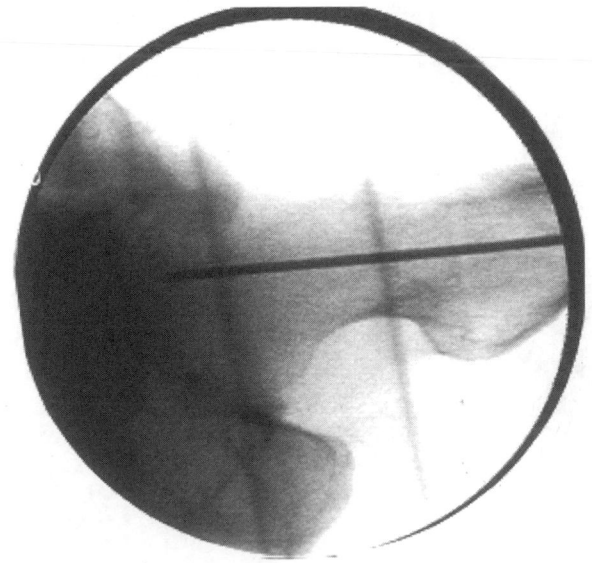

Figure 14.2 *X-ray image of lateral hip with pin in place.*

15. HIP SCREW AP VIEW
(PATIENT IN LATERAL POSITION)

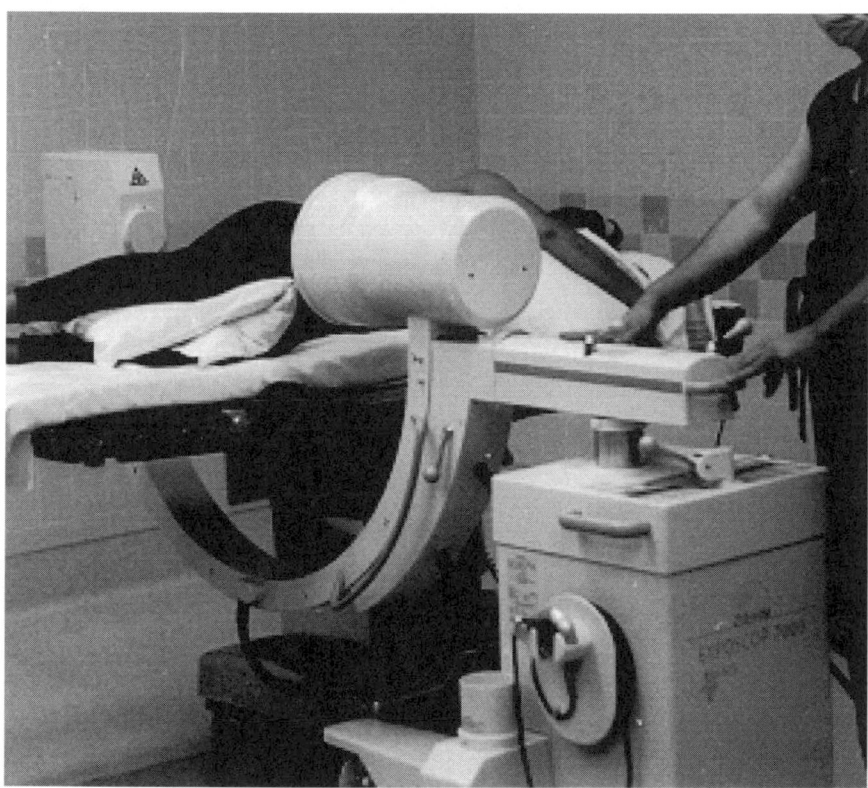

PATIENT POSITION: Patient will be in lateral position with the affected hip up.

C-ARM POSITION: C-arm will enter in the perpendicular to patient then rotate underneath to the ap projection.

Notes: In the ap projection c-arm may have to be tilted to view head of femur.

Angle c-arm to view hip in a true ap plane.

Pelvis program on c-arm better illustrates these images.

Figure 15.1 *C-arm in ap projection of affected hip.*

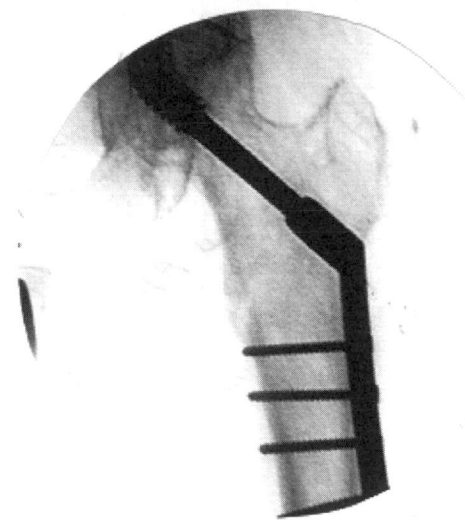

Figure 15.2 *X-ray image of ap hip with instrumentation.*

16. HIP SCREW LATERAL VIEW
(PATIENT IN LATERAL POSITION)

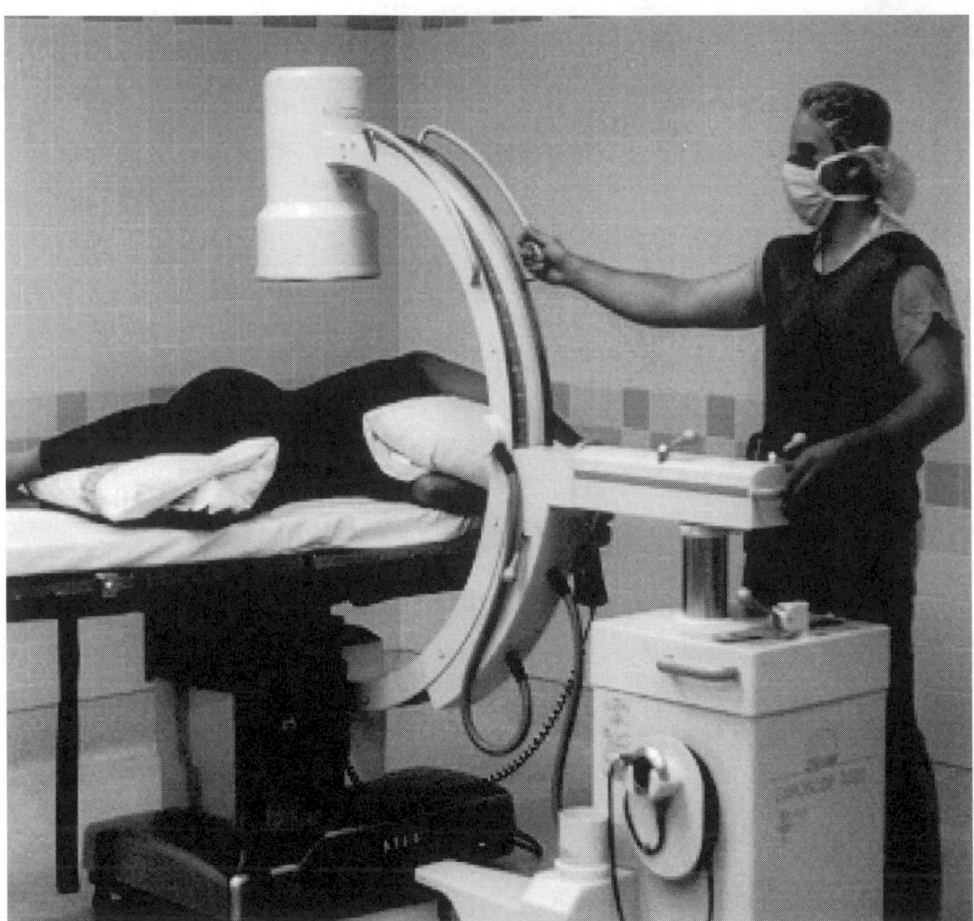

PATIENT POSITION:
Patient will be in lateral position with the affected hip up.

C-ARM POSITION:
C-arm will enter in the perpendicular to patient and in the lateral position.

Notes: C-arm may have to be rotated over or backward to unalign femurs.

Physician will generally stand posterior to the patient.

Ensure not to bump instrumentation protruding from hip.

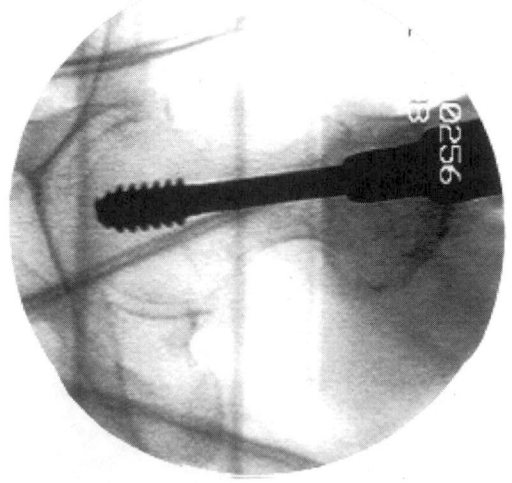

Figure 16.2 *X-ray image of lateral hip with instrumentation.*

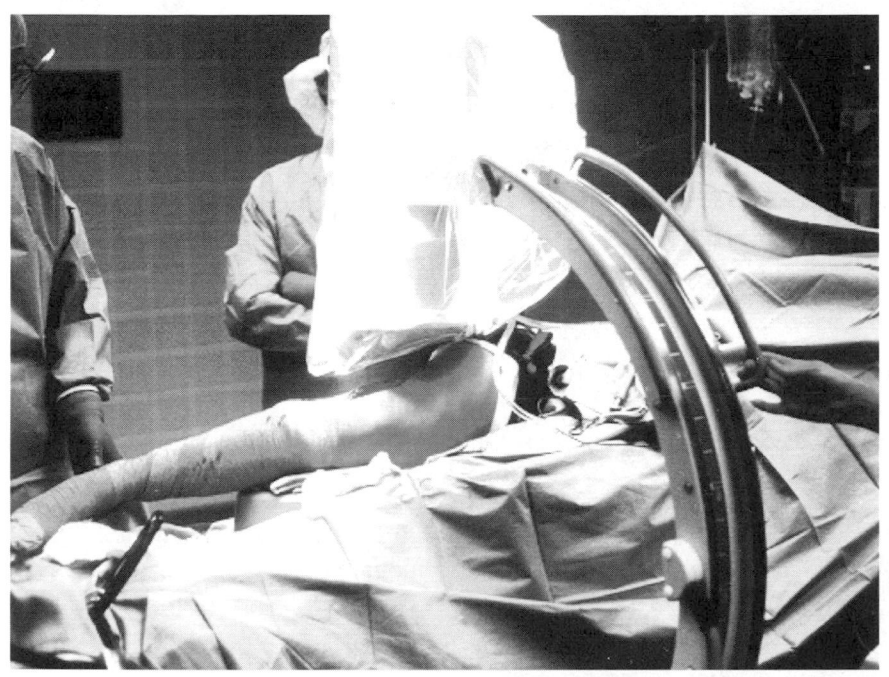

Figure 16.3 *The c-arm in the lateral projection of the femur. Note how the knee is positioned with assistance to promote a true lateral of the femur.*

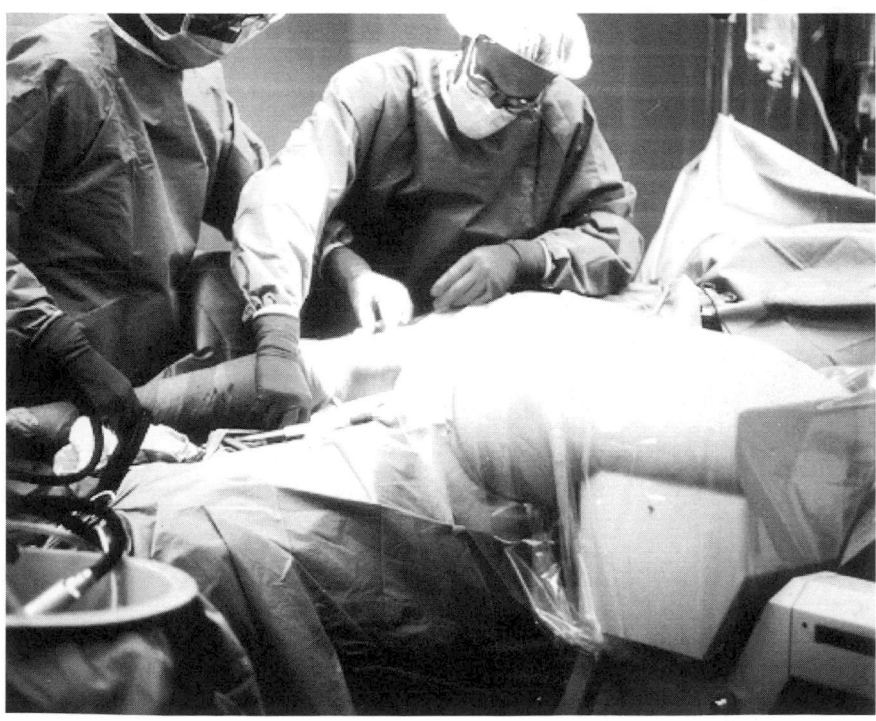

Figure 16.4 *The c-arm rotated underneath the table to view the ap of the hip and femur during a hip screw procedure.*

17. HIP ARTHROSCOPY
(PATIENT IN SUPINE POSITION)

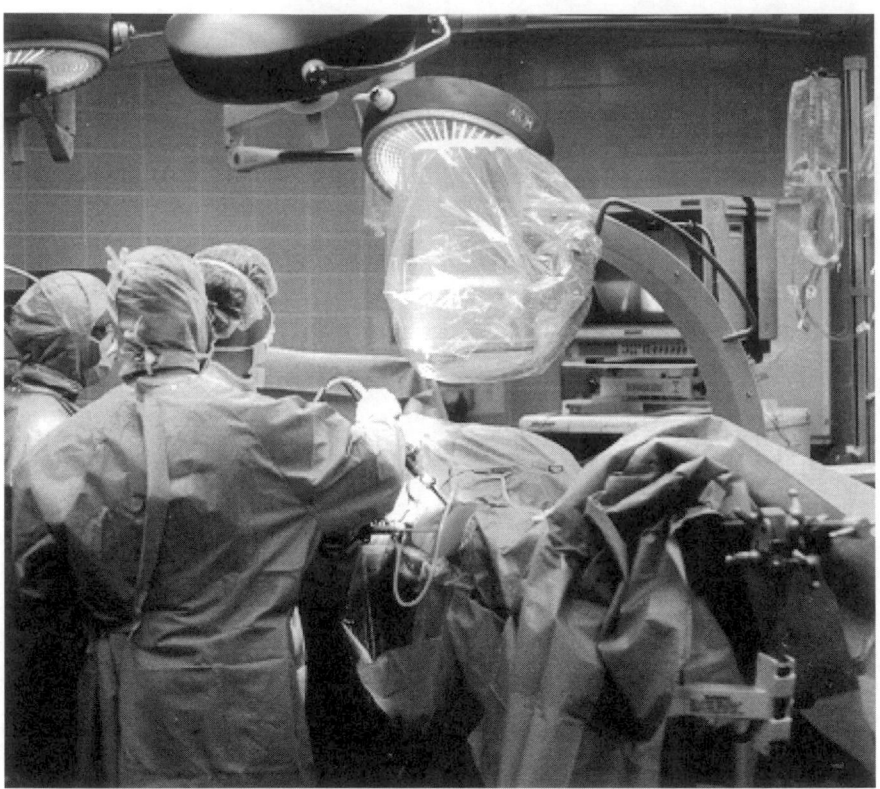

Figure 17.1 *C-arm in ap projection of affected hip.*

PATIENT POSITION: Patient will be supine with legs abducted to physician's preference.

C-ARM POSITION: C-arm will enter perpendicular to patient in the ap projection and on opposite side of physician.

Notes: C-arm may have to be manipulated over or backward to obtain clear views of the femoral head and acetabulum.

Rotating the c-arm backward 5 to 7 degrees along with a 2- to 6-degree cephalad tilt will give Crutcher's View of the hip.

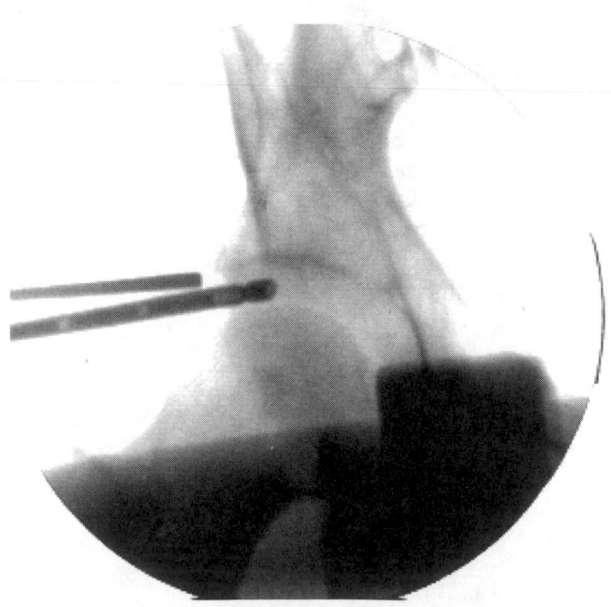

Figure 17.2 *X-ray image of ap hip with scope inserted.*

18. HIP ARTHROSCOPY
(PATIENT IN LATERAL POSITION)

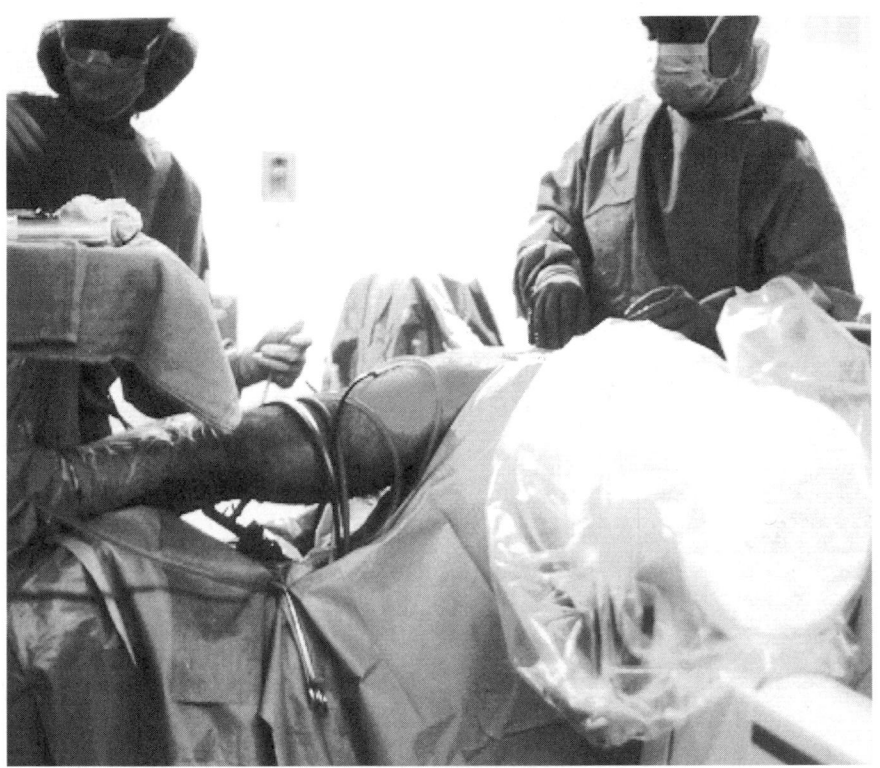

Figure 18.1 *C-arm in ap projection of affected hip.*

PATIENT POSITION: Patient will be in the lateral position with the affected hip up.

C-ARM POSITION: C-arm will enter perpendicular to patient in the ap projection, showing the lateral view of the hip. Rotate c-arm underneath table to view the ap of the hip.

Notes: Place image intensifier close to the patient to create a larger field of view.

Ensure not to bump instrumentation when moving the c-arm form the ap to the lateral position.

C-arm should be positioned perpendicular to the patient's hip to view a true ap of the affected hip.

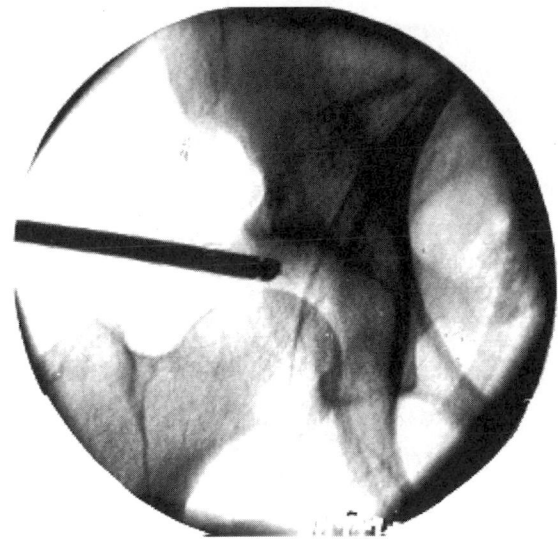

Figure 18.2 *X-ray image of affected hip.*

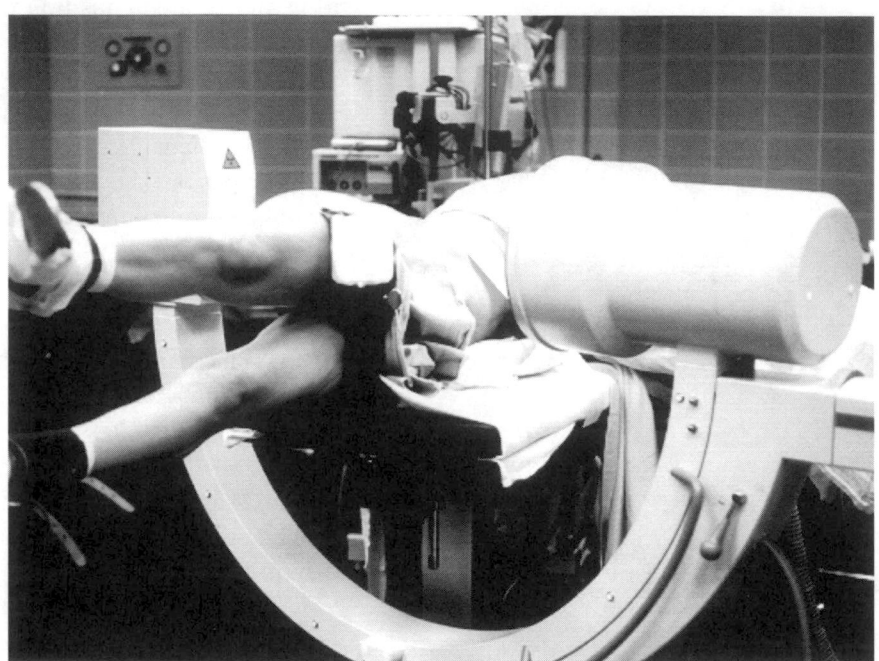

Figure 18.3 *Patient in the lateral position with the c-arm rotated underneath the table to view the ap of the hip.*

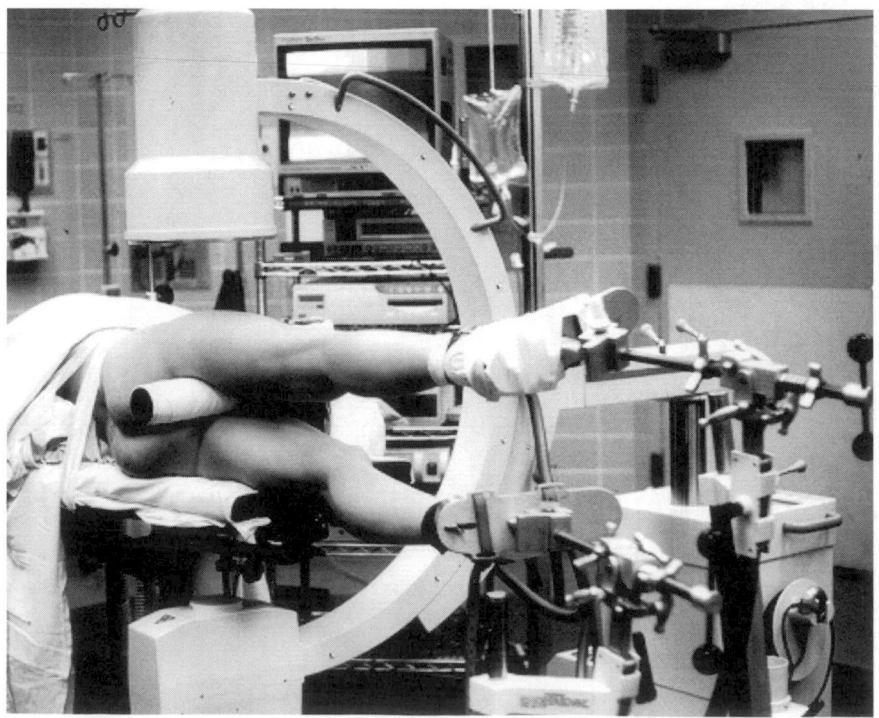

Figure 18.4 *C-arm showing the lateral view of the affected hip. Use the Crutcher's view to show a better aspect of the hip.*

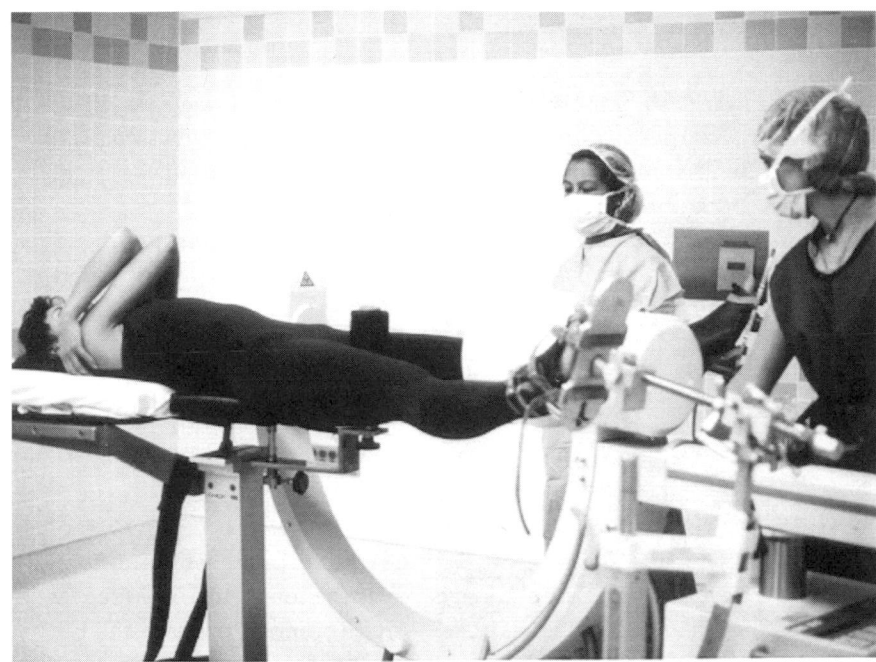

Figure 8.5 *When the patient is positioned supine during a hip arthroscopy and the lateral view is desired, the c-arm may have to be manipulated between the legs then rotated underneath to obtain the lateral view.*

19. HIP OSTEOTOMY

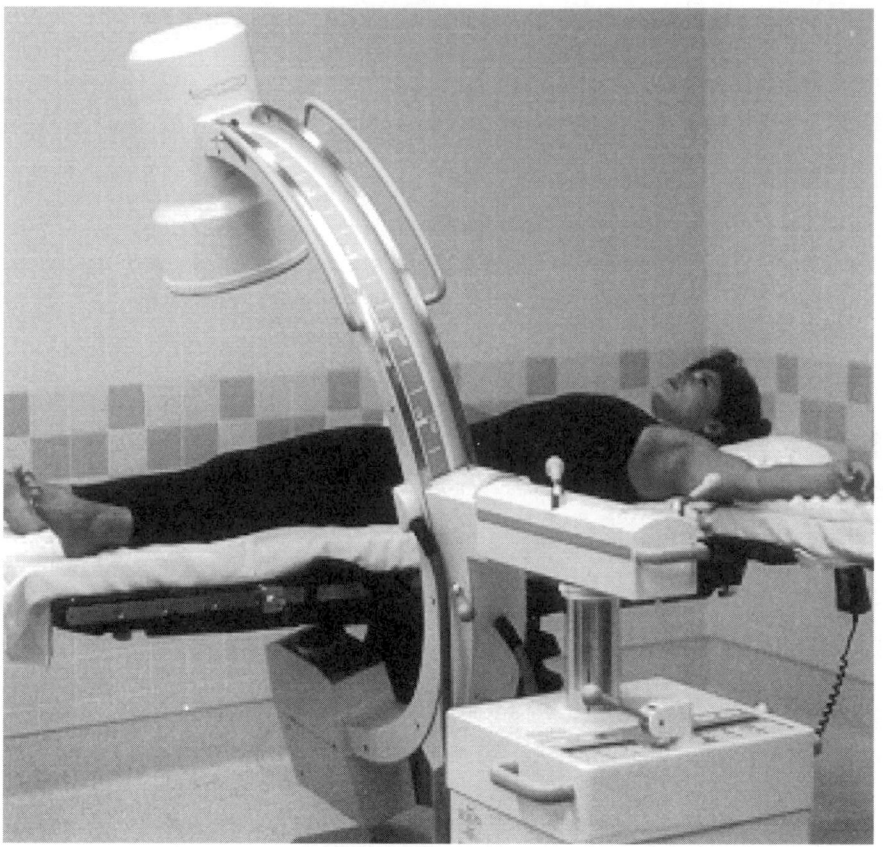

PATIENT POSITION: Patient will be supine with the legs extended or the affected hip slightly flexed.

C-ARM POSITION: C-arm will enter in the ap projection perpendicular to the patient.

Notes: Cover c-arm with sterile drape when working over sterile field.

C-arm may have to be tilted or rotated to acquire the desired view.

Angling the c-arm five to seven degrees cephalad and rotating over the top 8 to 15 degrees will give Toomey's view of the hip.

Figure 19.1   *C-arm in ap projection of the hip.*

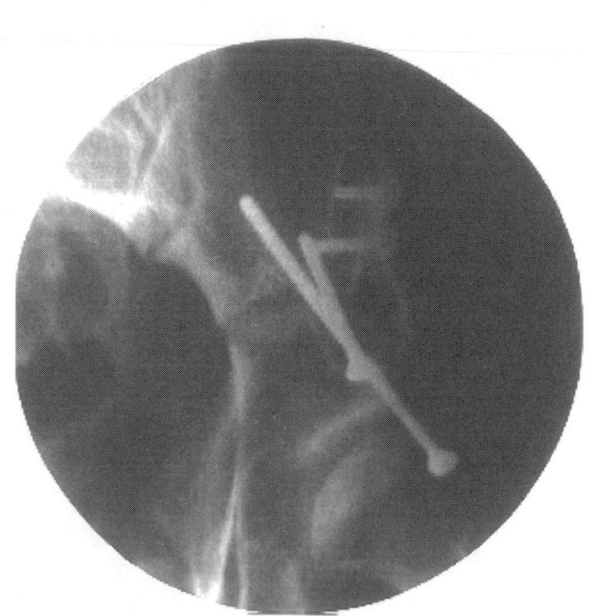

Figure 19.2   *X-ray image of hip with instrumentation.*

20. TOTAL HIP REVISION

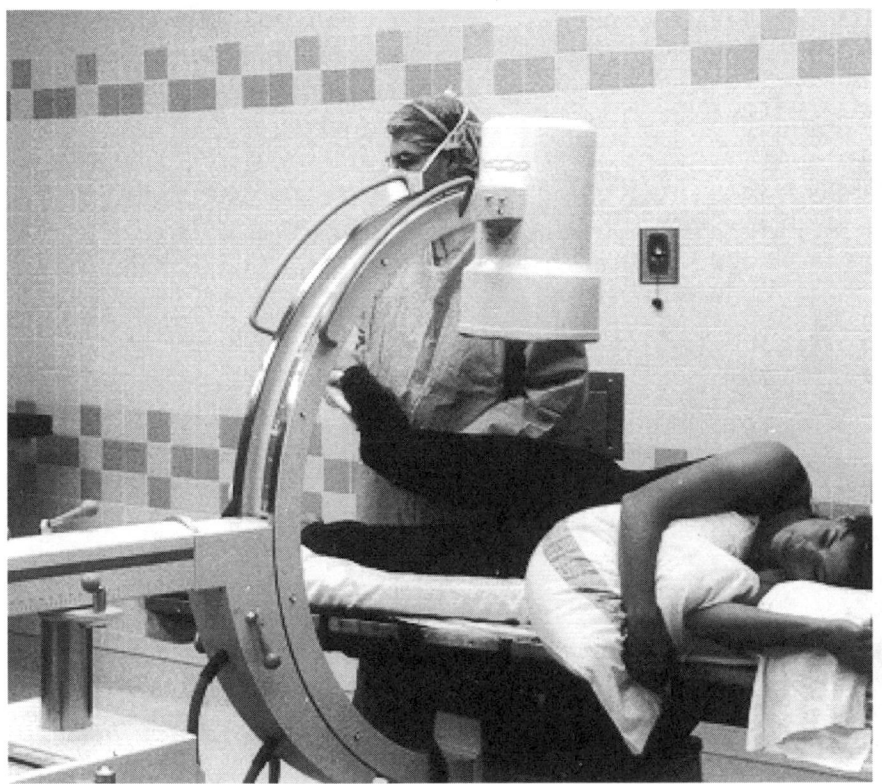

Figure 20.1 *C-arm in lateral projection with hip dislocated.*

PATIENT POSITION: Patient is usually positioned on the side with legs scissored and the affected hip up.

C-ARM POSITION: C-arm will enter opposite side of physician to view affected hip. C-arm will be in ap position.

Notes: Doctor will stand posterior to affected hip.

It may be necessary to roll c-arm over the top to throw the unaffected hip out of the view.

Doctor or assistant will rotate leg to create ap and lateral view.

Rotation of the leg 30 to 45 degrees will give Wilson's ridge of femoral neck.

Preoperative fluoroscopy should be used to determine adequate visualization of entire affected area.

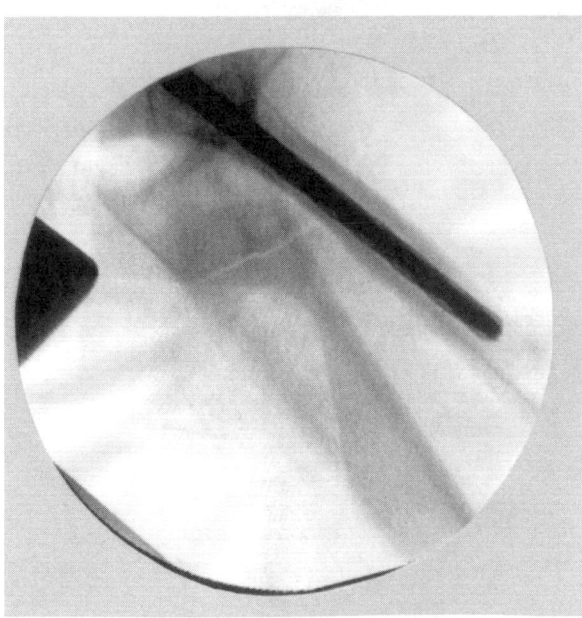

Figure 20.2 *C-arm image of femur during revision with reamer inserted.*

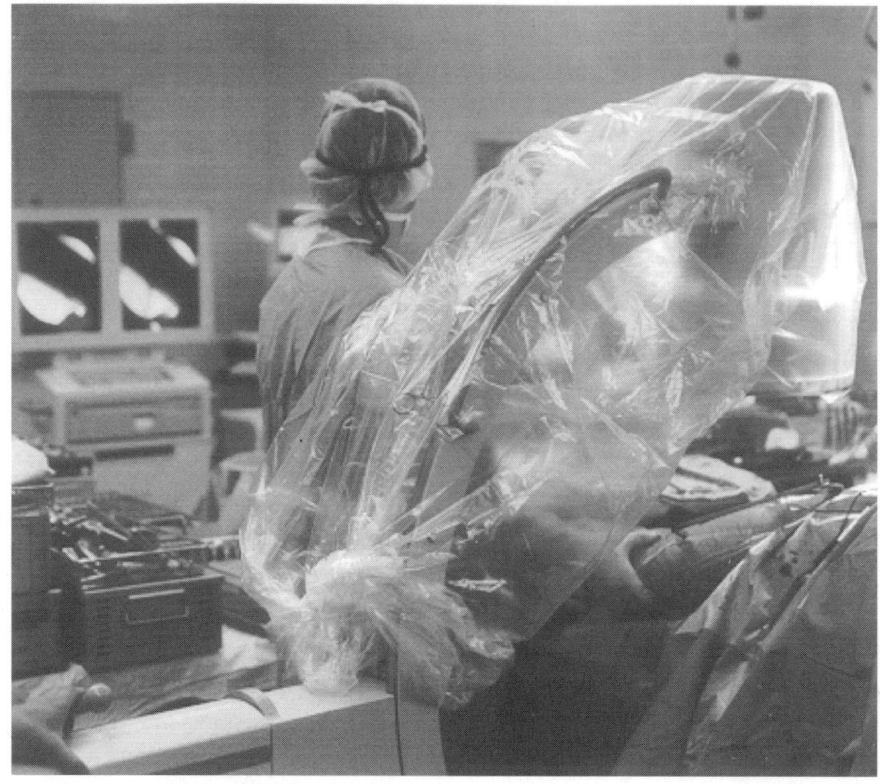

Figure 20.3 *When obtaining a lateral view of the femur during a hip revision, the assistant rotates the leg downward to promote a lateral image.*

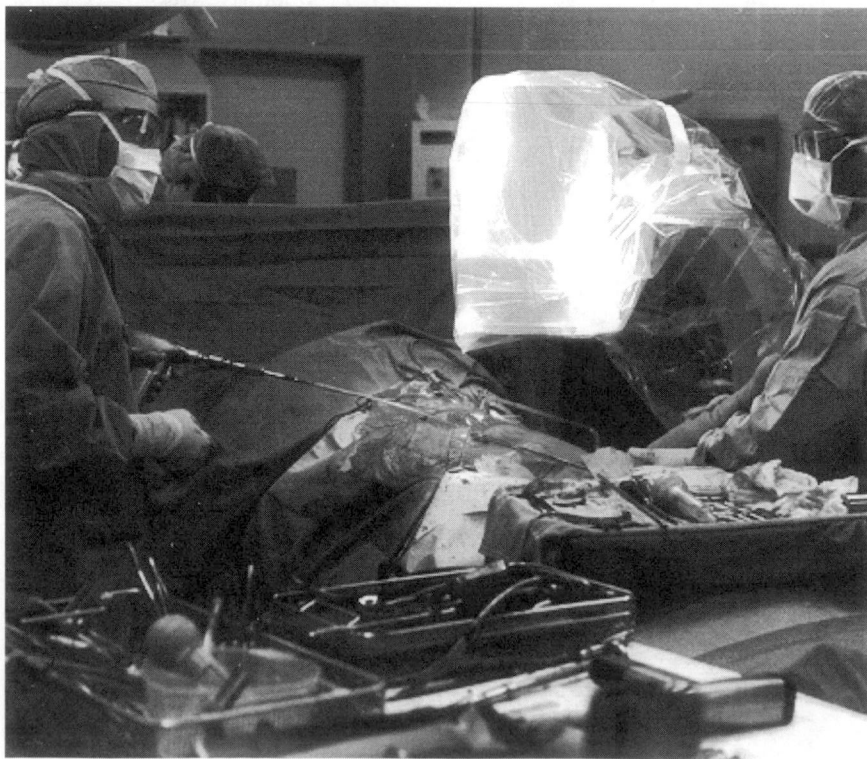

Figure 20.4 *The assistant has rotated the leg so the foot is skyward. This dislocates the hip and shows a pa image.*

21. ACETABULAR/PELVIC FRACTURE

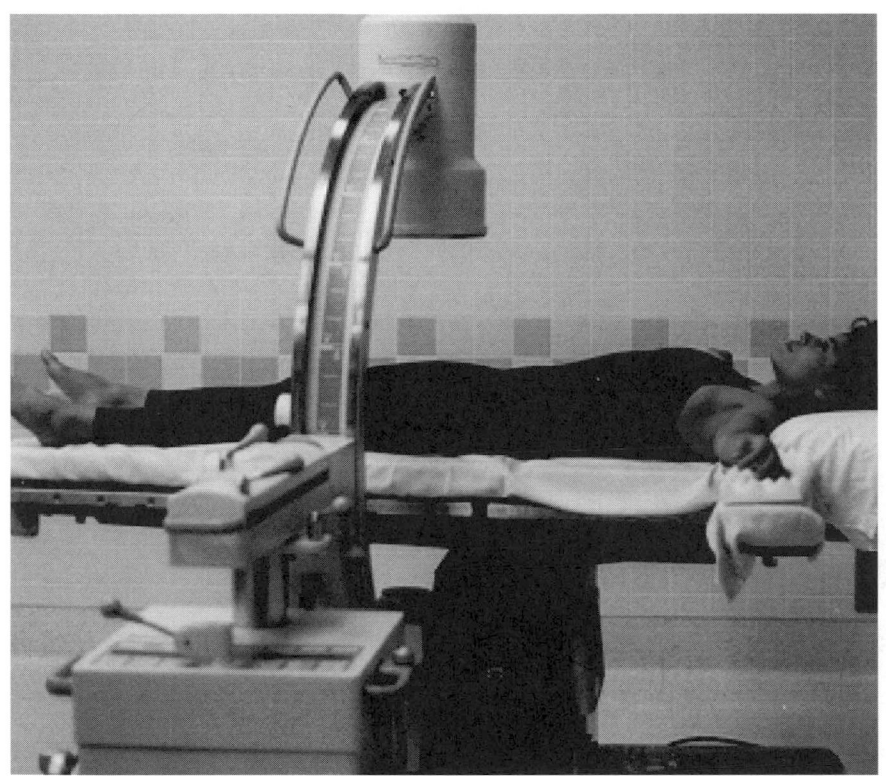

Figure 21.1 *C-arm in ap projection of pelvis.*

PATIENT POSITION: Patient will be supine or with the affected acetabular in the left posterior oblique (LPO) or right posterior oblique (RPO) position. Patient may be prone if fracture is in acetabular region.

C-ARM POSITION: C-arm will face the patient in the ap projection.

Notes: C-arm may have to be tilted over or backwards to view acetabulum or pelvis in the Judeau views.

C-arm may have to be angled cephalad or caudal to view inlet and outlet views.

Pelvis program on c-arm better illustrates these views.

Ensure area underneath table is clear to allow movement of the c-arm.

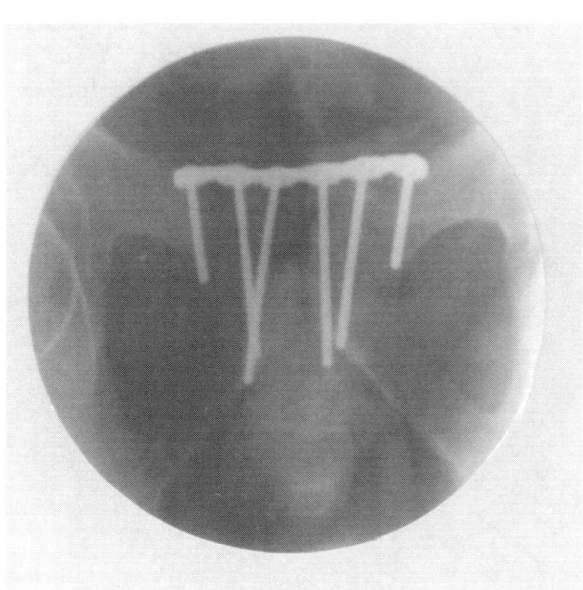

Figure 21.2 *C-arm image of pelvis with instrumentation.*

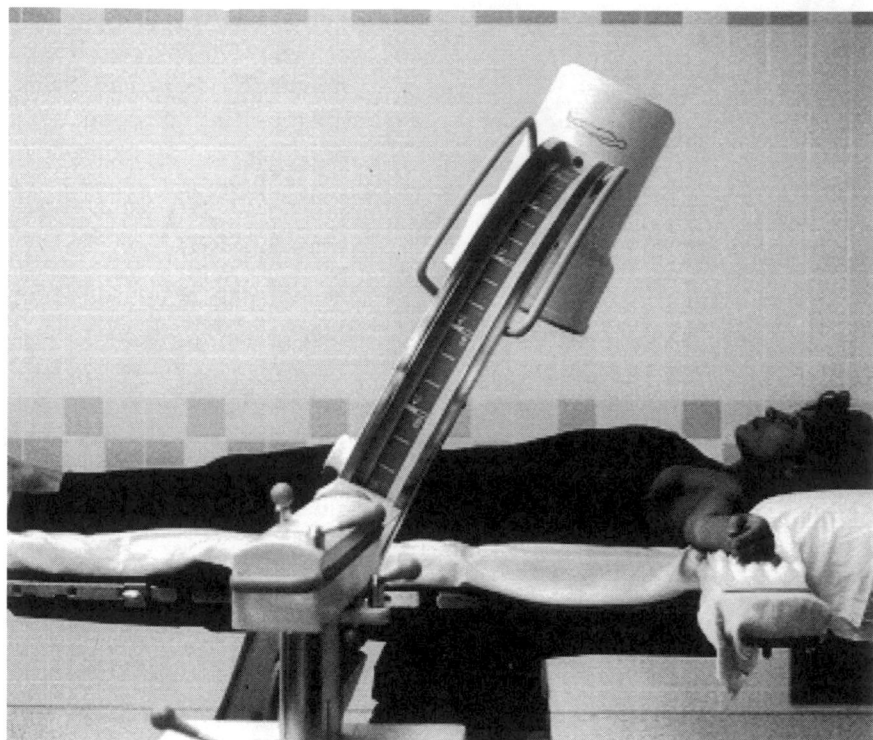

Figure 21.3 *During pelvis or pubic fractures, the inlet and outlet views may be otained by angling the c-arm caudal or cephalad.*

The patient is supine with the c-arm angled caudal to obtain the outlet view.

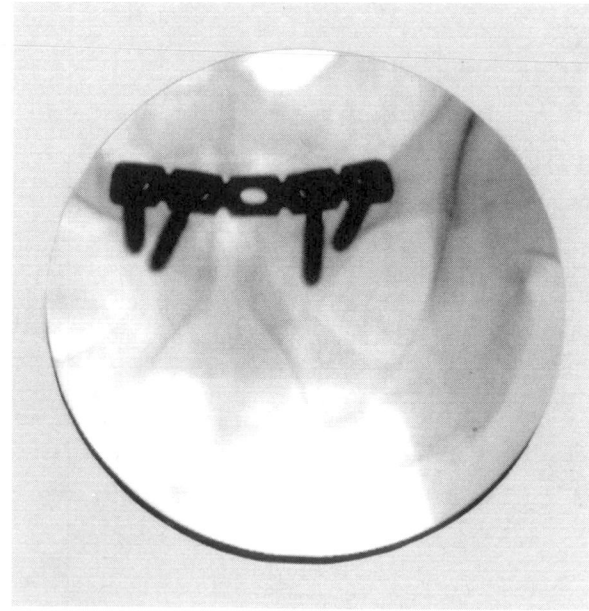

Figure 21.4 *X-ray image of the outlet view.*

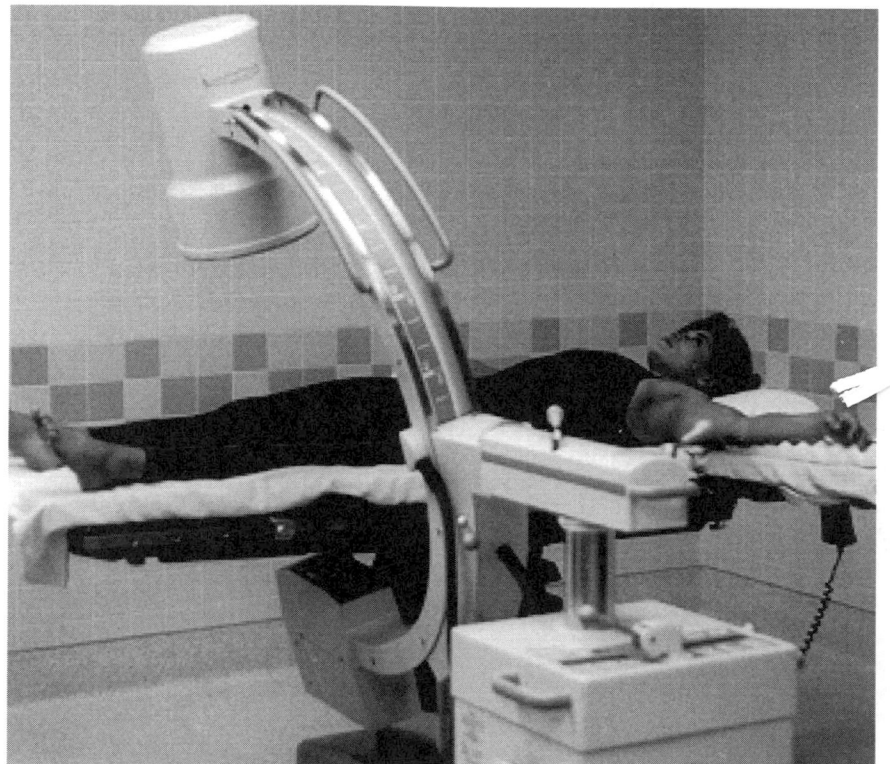

Figure 21.5 *The patient is supine with the c-arm angled cephalad to obtain the inlet view.*

Note that if the patient is in the oblique position the c-arm will have to be rotated over or backward to align with the pelvis.

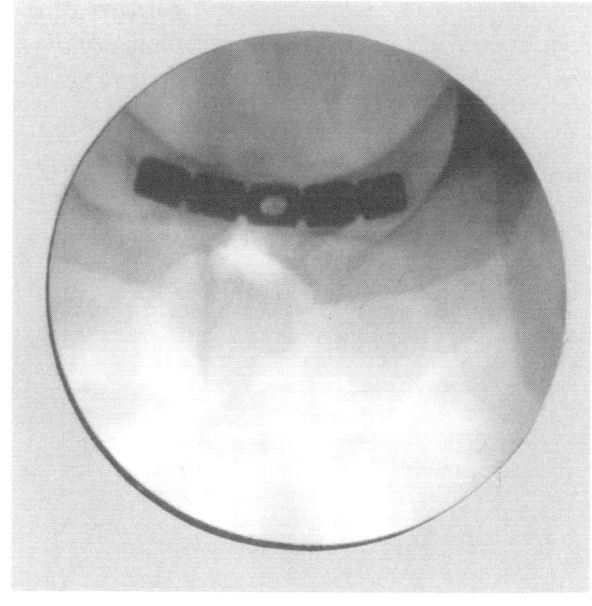

Figure 21.6 *X-ray image of the inlet view.*

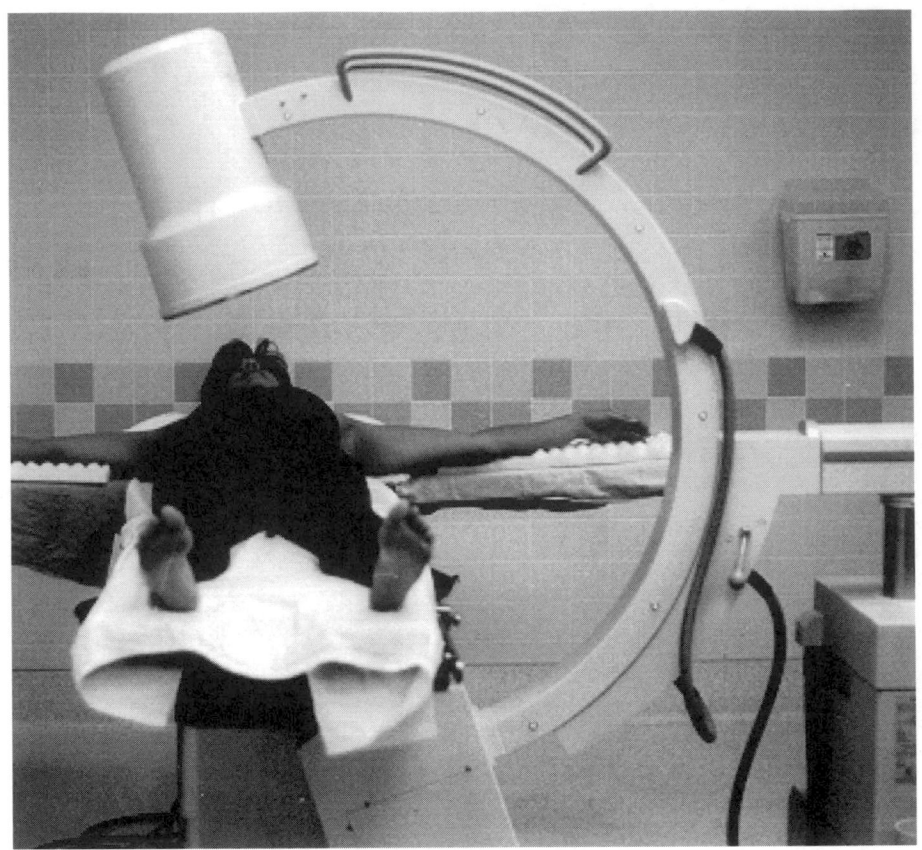

Figure 21.7 *The patient is supine with the c-arm rotated over to view the oblique hip.*

During fixation of pelvis and acetabulum fractures, the oblique or "Judeau" views are obtained by rotating the c-arm over or backward to the desired angle.

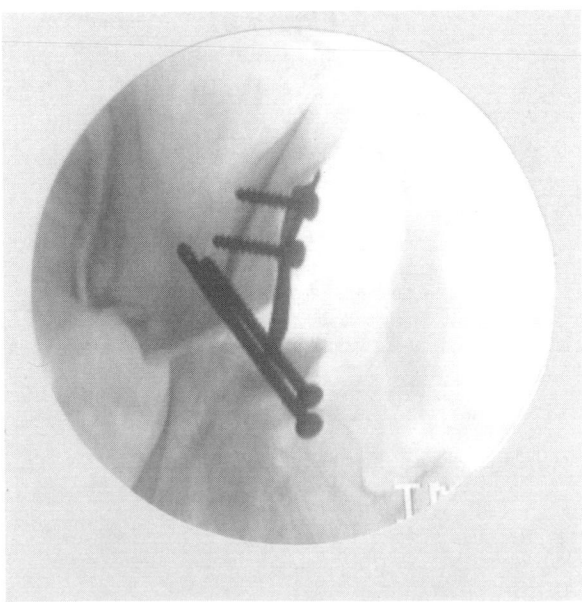

Figure 21.8 *X-ray image of the hip with instrumentation inserted.*

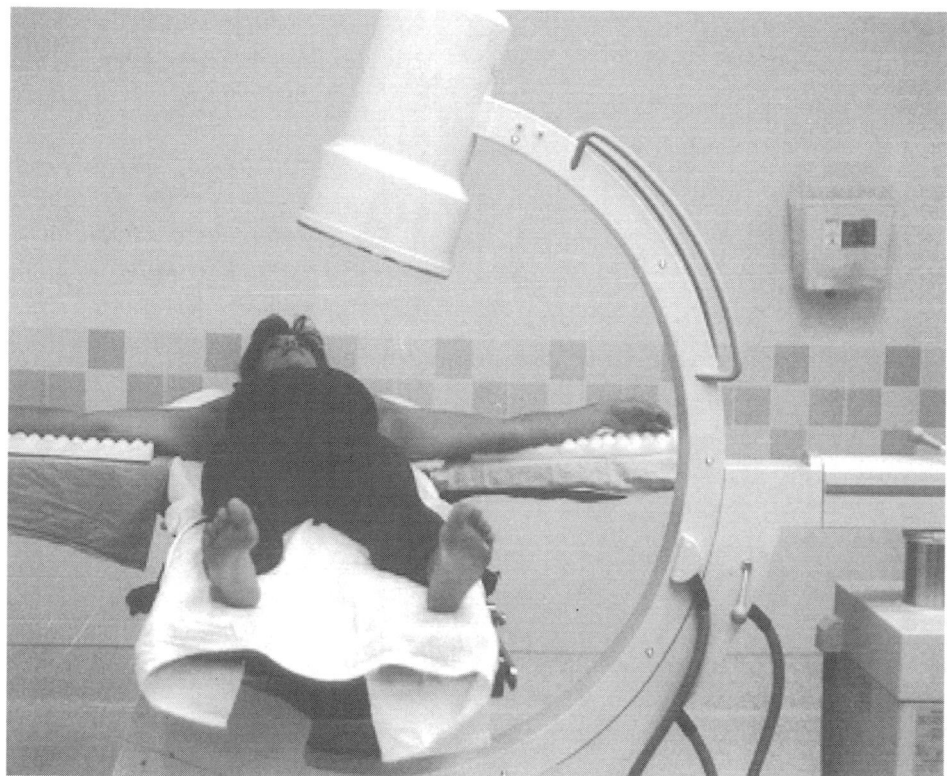

Figure 21.9 *The patient is supine with the c-arm rotated backward to view the oblique hip.*

Note that if the patient is in the oblique position, the c-arm should enter in the straight pa projection.

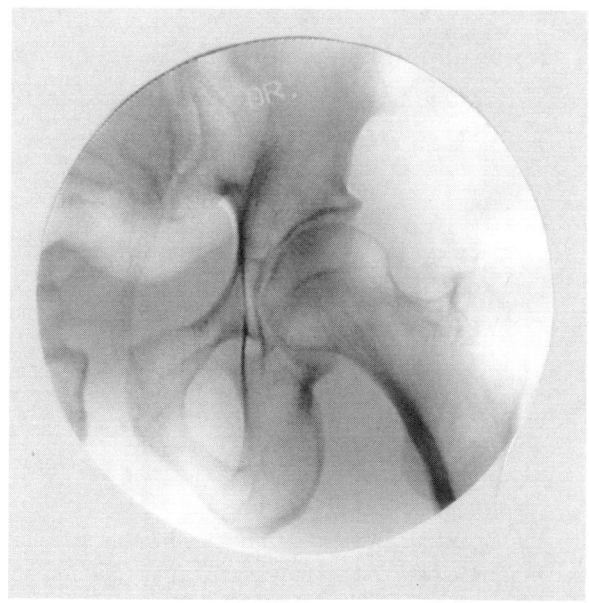

Figure 21.10 *X-ray image of the affected hip.*

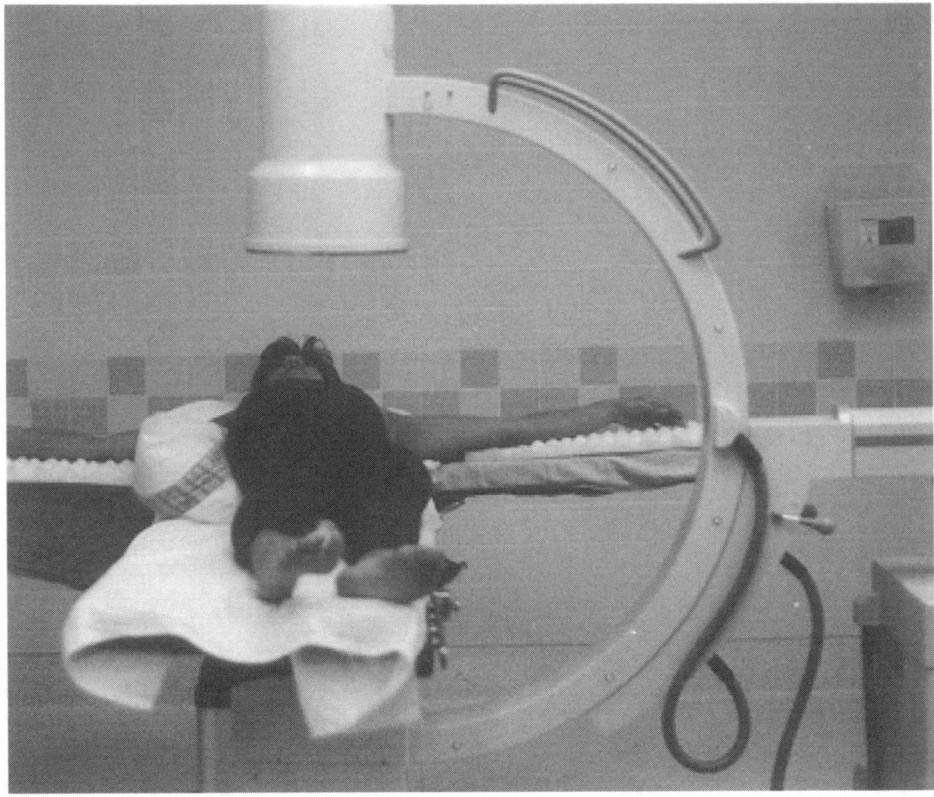

Figure 21.11 *The patient in the LPO position.*

Note that pelvis fractures may have to be repaired with the patient oblique and either supine or prone.

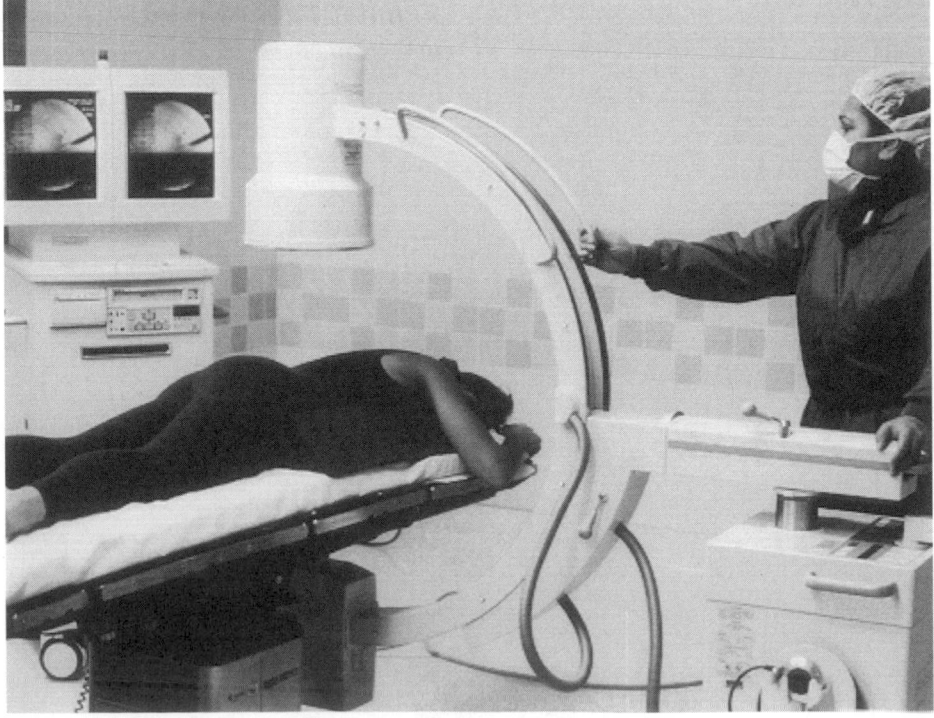

Figure 21.12 *The patient in the LAO position.*

22. TIBIAL OSTEOTOMY

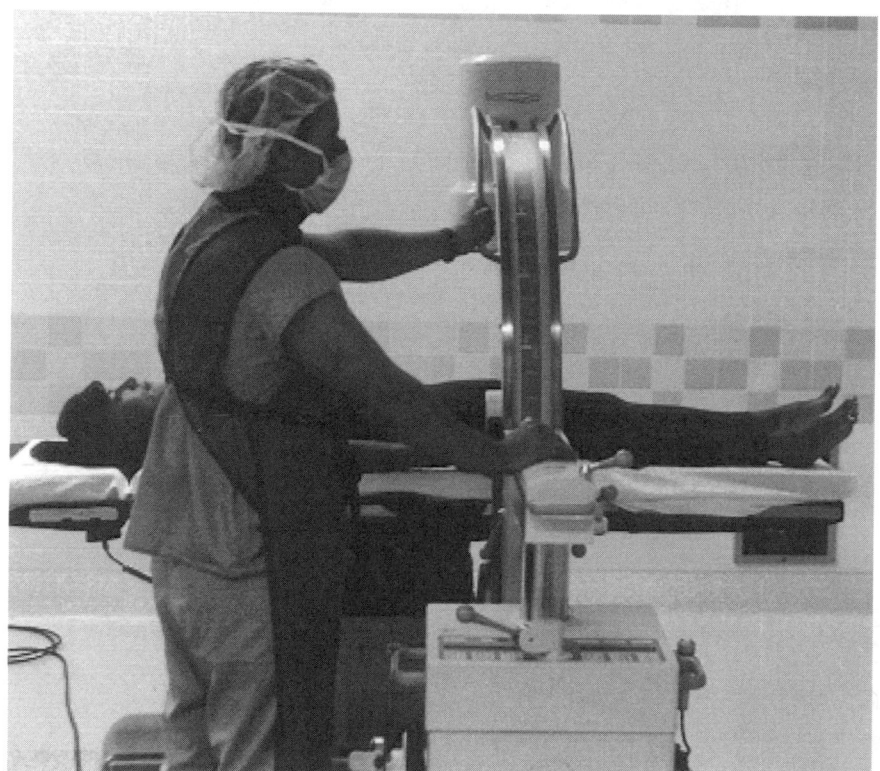

PATIENT POSITION: Patient will be supine with knee on radiolucent portion of table.

C-ARM POSITION: C-arm will enter in the ap projection centered over the affected knee.

Notes: Lower c-arm to create a larger field of view.

C-arm may have to be tilted or rotated to create a true ap view of knee.

Cover c-arm with sterile drape before positioning over patient.

Figure 22.1 *C-arm in ap projection of knee.*

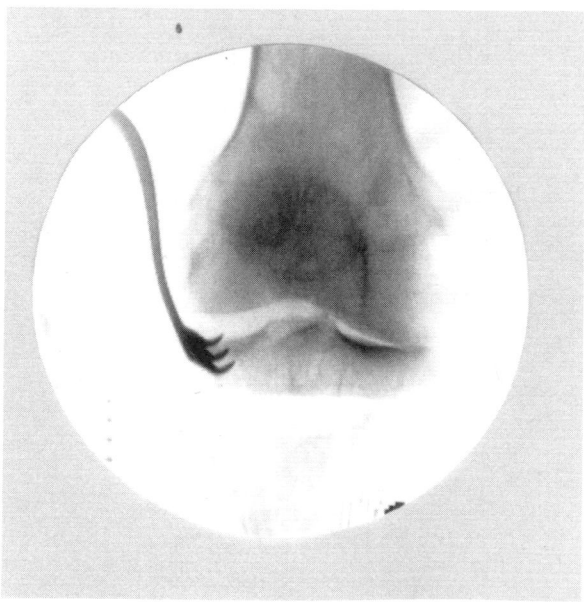

Figure 22.2 *X-ray image of ap knee with osteotomy cut.*

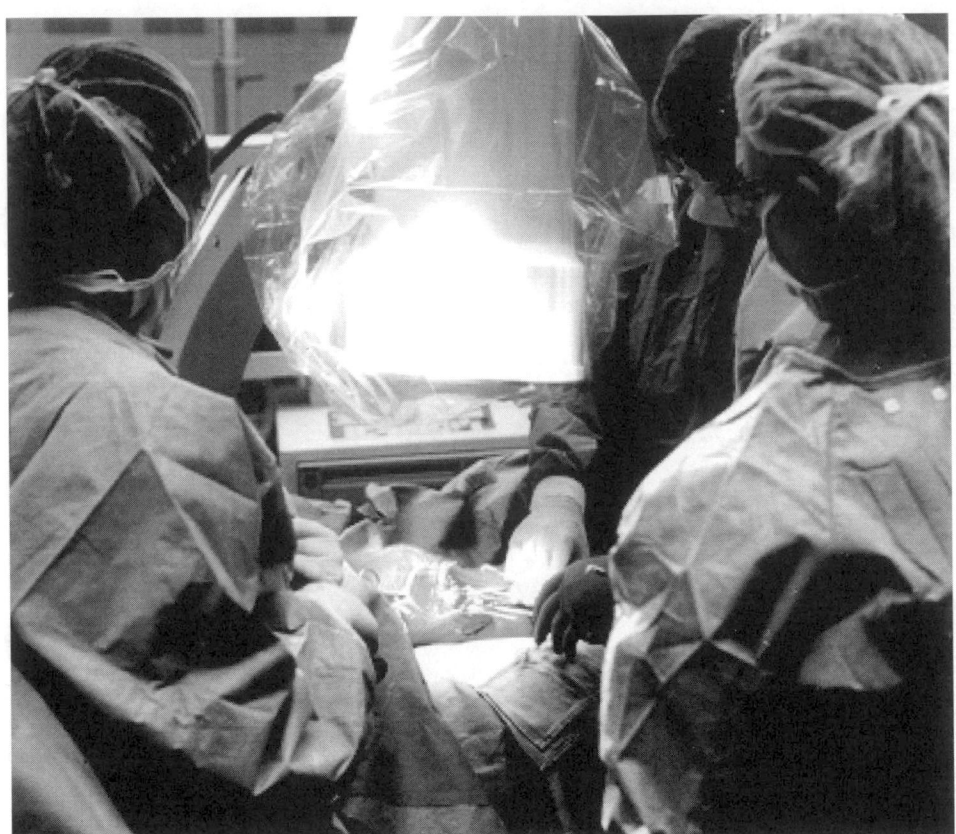

Figure 22.3 *During tibial osteotomy, lower the c-arm close to the leg. It is important to see a larger field of view to help with proper alignment.*

23. DISTAL TIBIAL OSTEOMTOMY
(AP VIEW)

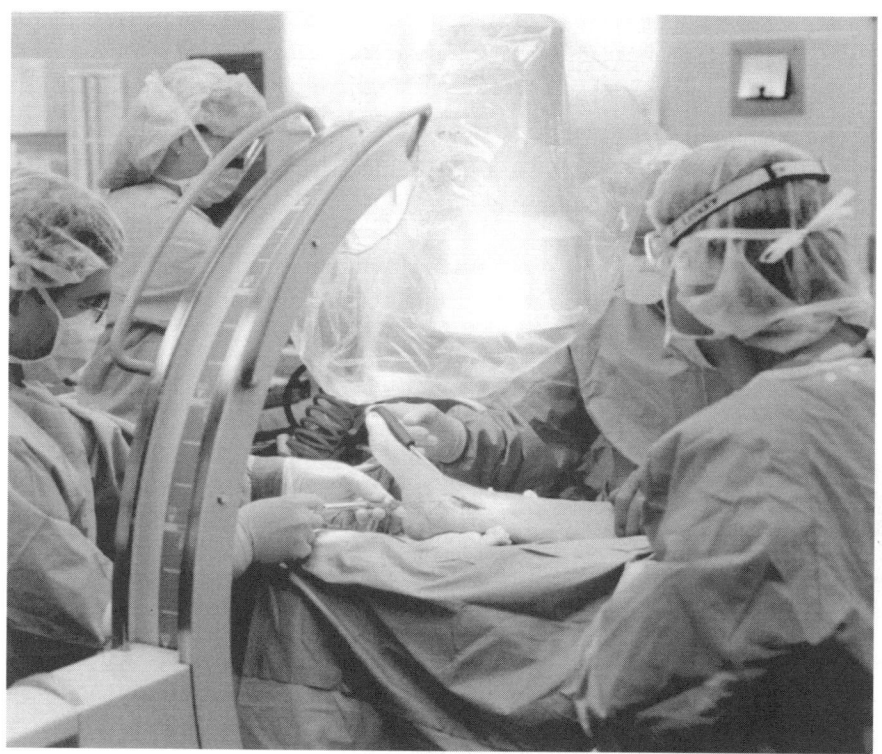

PATIENT POSITION: Patient will be supine with legs on radiolucent portion of the table.

C-ARM POSITION: C-arm will enter perpendicular to the patient and in the ap projection.

Notes: C-arm should be covered with sterile drape before positioning over sterile field.

C-arm may have to be tilted over or backward to obtain a true ap of the ankle joint.

Position image intensifier close to the ankle to present a larger field of view.

Figure 23.1 *C-arm in ap view of affected tibia.*

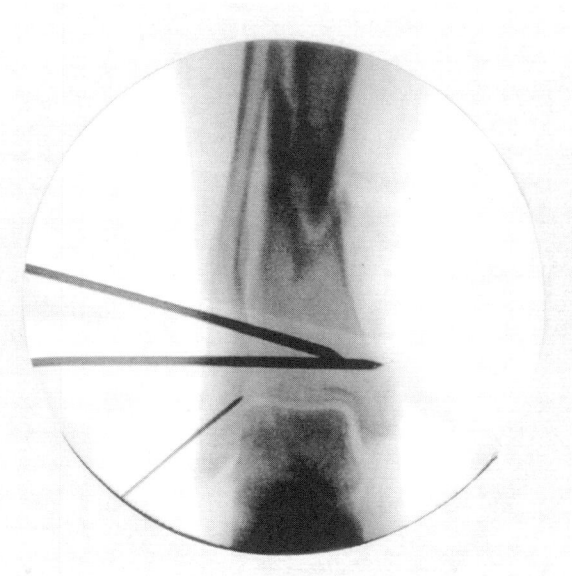

Figure 23.2 *X-ray image of affected tibia.*

24. POSTERIOR CRUCIATE LIGAMENT REPAIR

(AP POSITION)

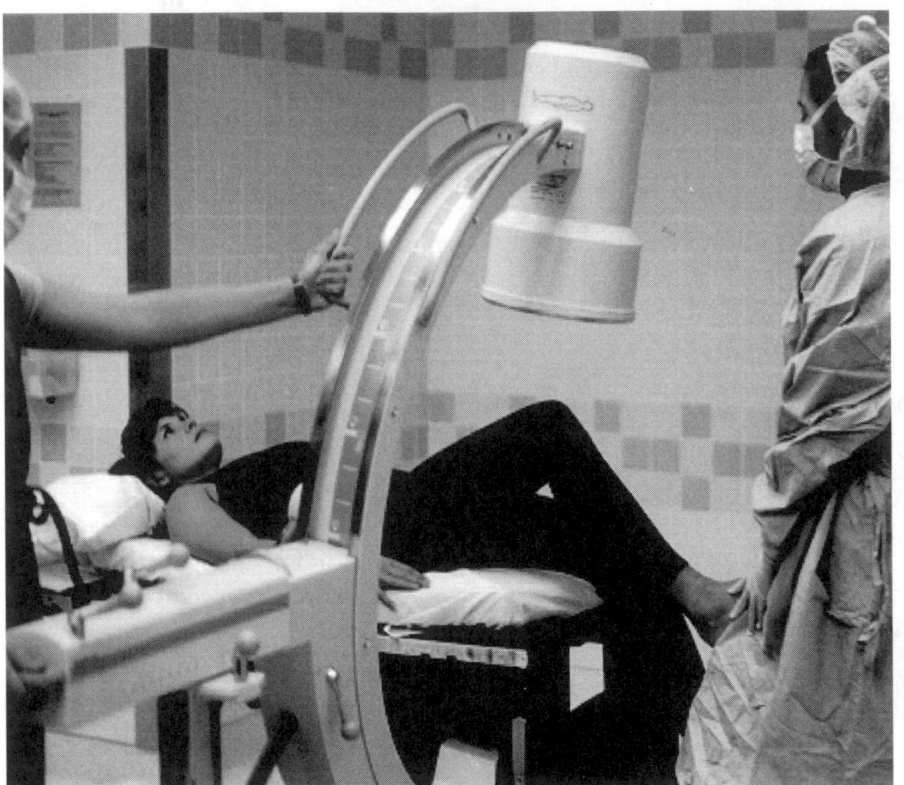

PATIENT POSITION:
Patient will be supine and positioned on arthroscopy table with affected knee bent.

C-ARM POSITION: C-arm will enter in the ap projection then rotate underneath to a lateral position.

Notes: Unaffected leg may have to be manipulated to allow entry of c-arm.

C-arm will have to be manipulated to create a true ap view.

Careful not to bump instrumentation when moving to ap view.

Figure 24. *C-arm in ap projection of affected knee.*

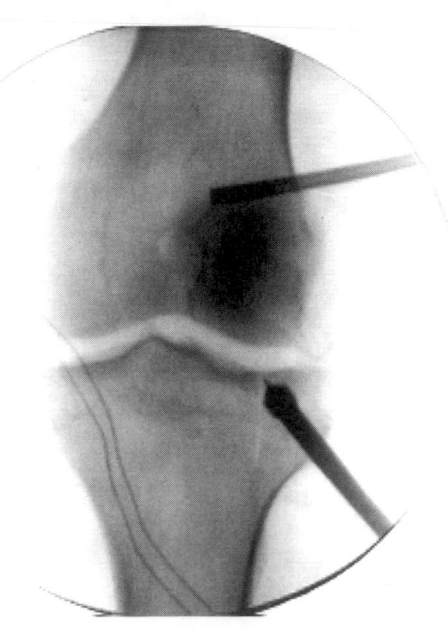

Figure 24.2 *X-ray image of ap knee with instrumentation.*

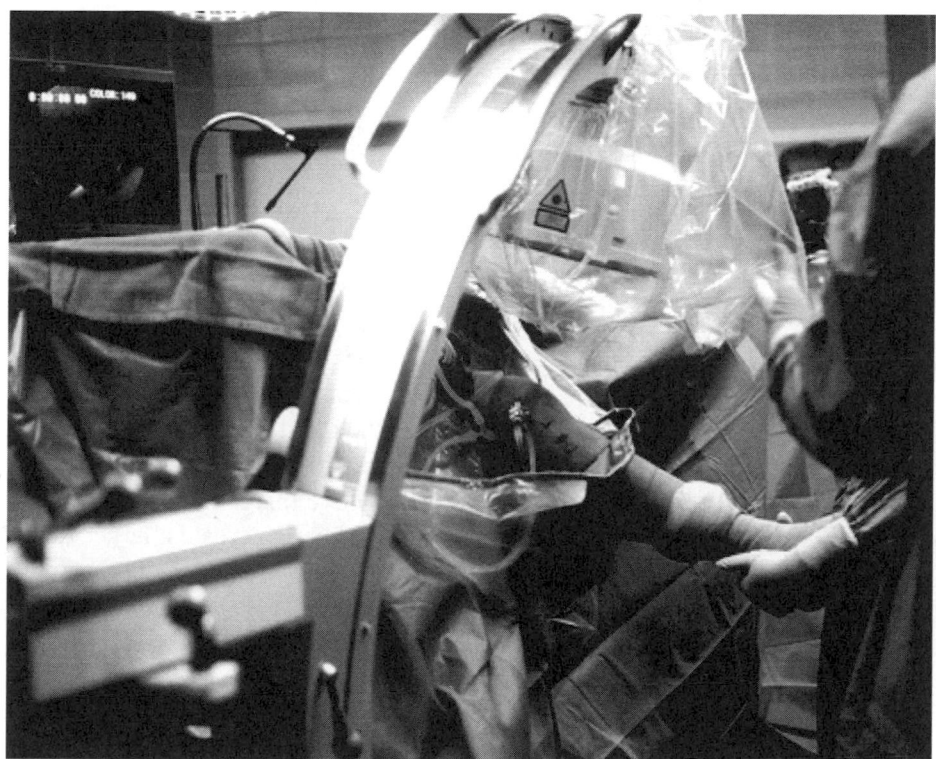

Figure 24.3 *This illustration shows the c-arm in the ap projection of the knee during a P.C.L. repair. The c-arm will have to be angled to align with the knee and show a true ap view.*

25. POSTERIOR CRUCIATE LIGAMENT REPAIR

(LATERAL POSITION)

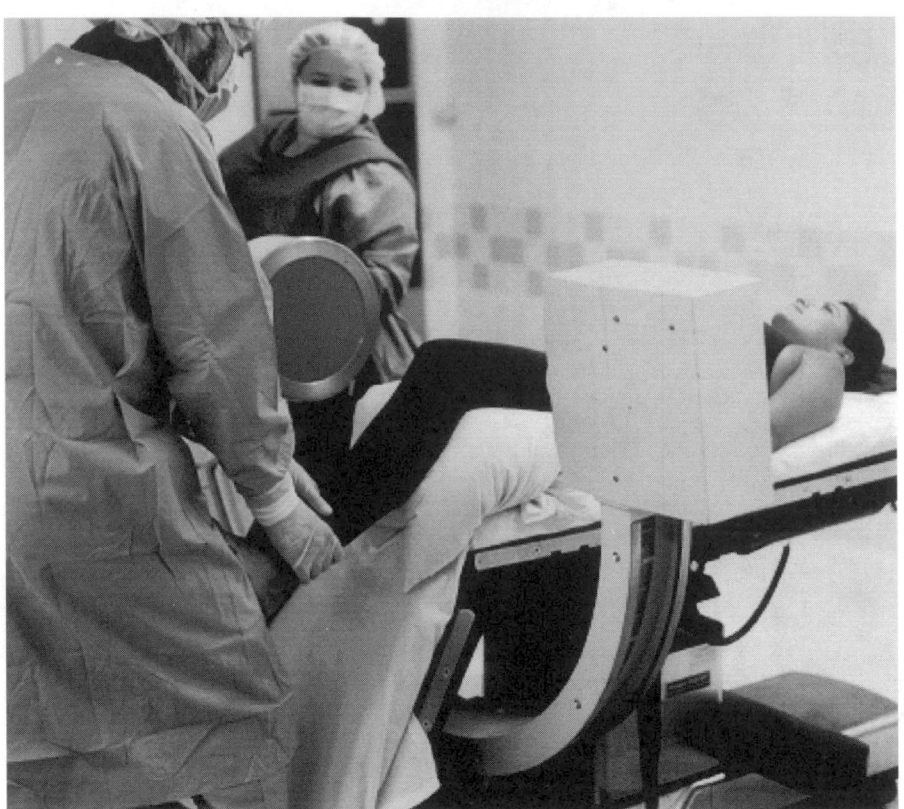

Figure 25.1 *C-arm in lateral projection of affected knee.*

PATIENT POSITION: Patient will be supine and positioned on arthroscopy table with affected knee bent.

C-ARM POSITION: C-arm will enter in the ap projection then rotate underneath to a lateral position.

Notes: C-arm may have to be tilted when in the lateral position to view distal femur. Move image intensifier close to knee to create a larger field of view.

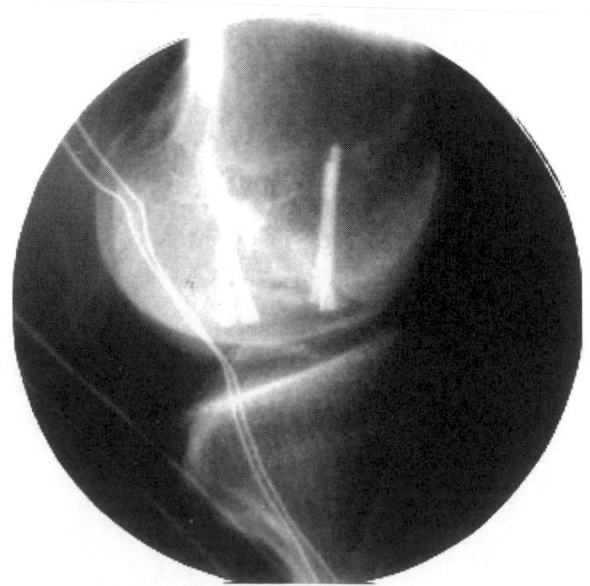

Figure 25.2 *X-ray image of lateral knee.*

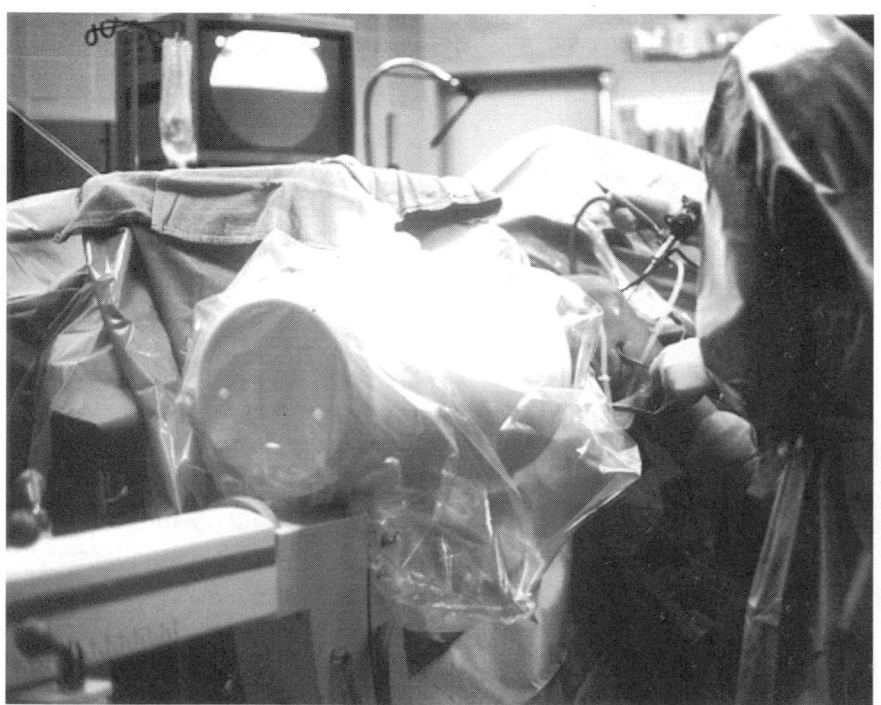

Figure 25.3 *The c-arm is rotated underneath the table to view the lateral of the knee. The c-arm may have to be angled to align with the knee to show a true lateral.*

26. ELBOW FRACTURE
(PATIENT SUPINE)

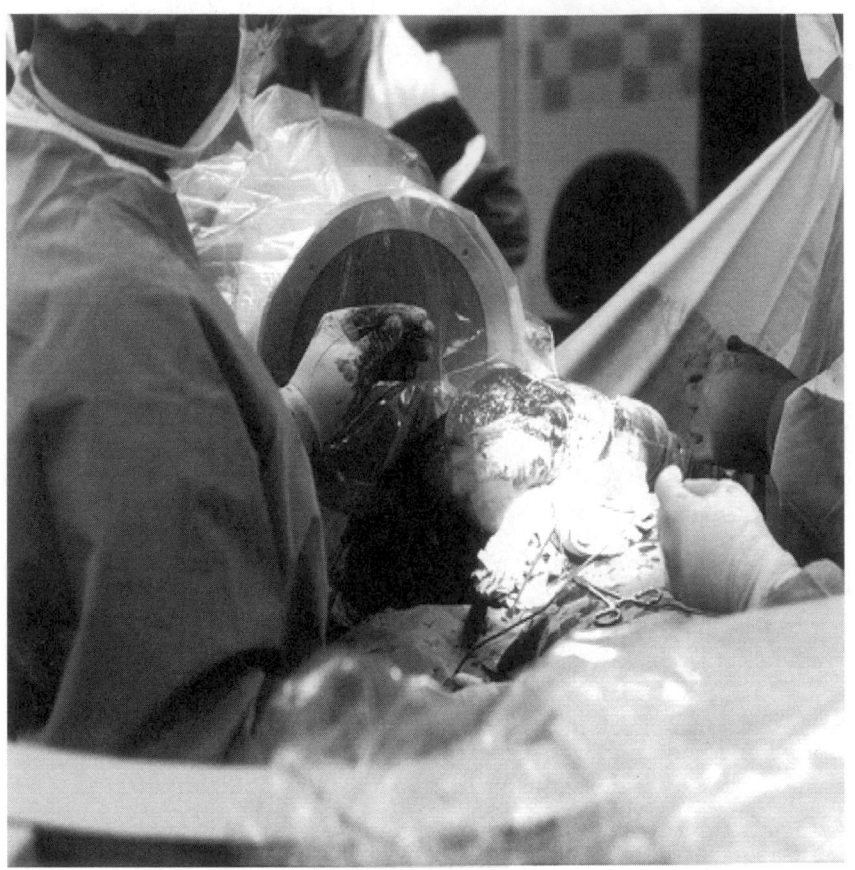

PATIENT POSITION: Patient will be supine with the affected arm across the chest area.

C-ARM POSITION: The c-arm will enter perpendicular to the patient. Tilt the c-arm to the position parallel to the floor.

Notes: Drape both ends of the c-arm when positioning over a sterile field.

Position the image intensifier close to the elbow for a larger field of view.

C-arm can be rotated circular to assist with obtaining the ap view.

Figure 26.1 *Patient and c-arm positioned for lateral view of the elbow.*

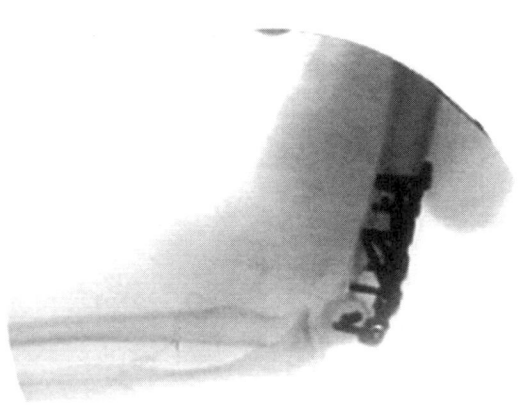

Figure 26.2 *X-ray image of the elbow with instrumentation.*

27. ELBOW FRACTURE
(PATIENT LATERAL)

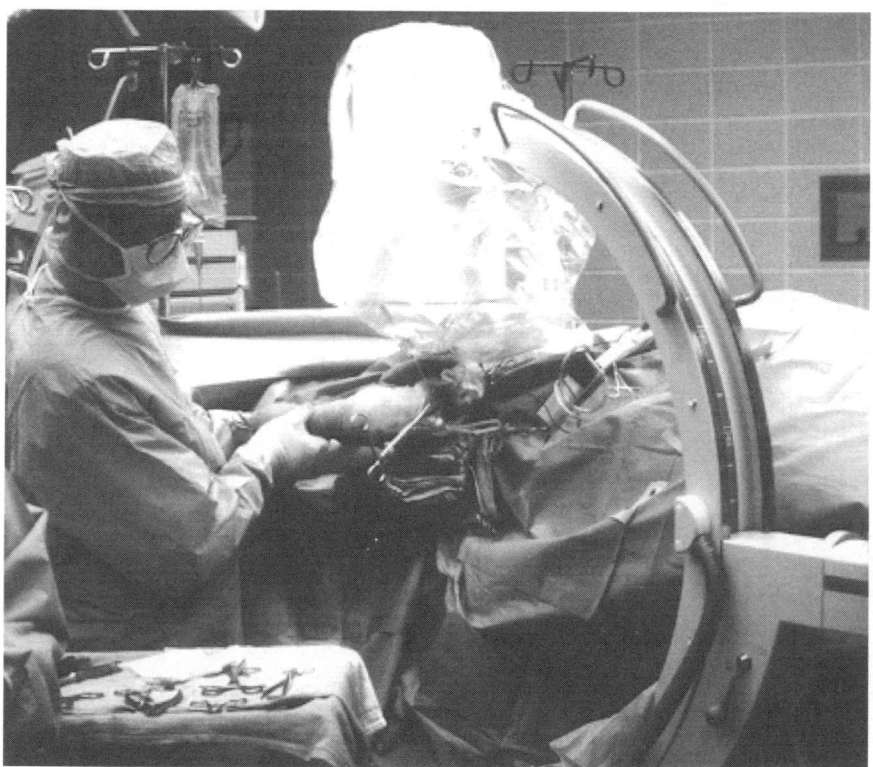

PATIENT POSITION: Patient will be lateral with the affected arm up and positioned down across the body.

C-ARM POSITION: C-arm will enter perpendicular to the patient and in the ap projection.

Notes: The c-arm will have to be manipulated to obtain true p.a. views.

Rotate the c-arm or the arm itself to view the lateral elbow.

Figure 27.1 *Patient and c-arm positioned for lateral view of the elbow.*

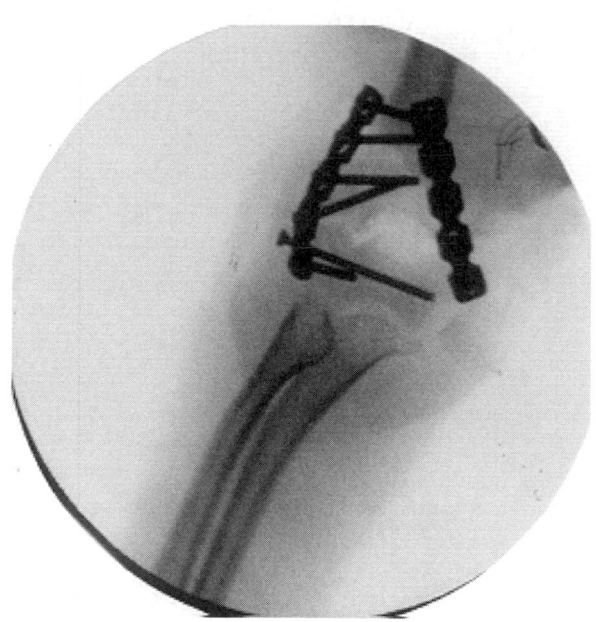

Figure 27.2 *X-ray image of the elbow with instrumentation.*

28. WRIST/FINGER PINNING
(USING FINGERTRAPS AP POSITION)

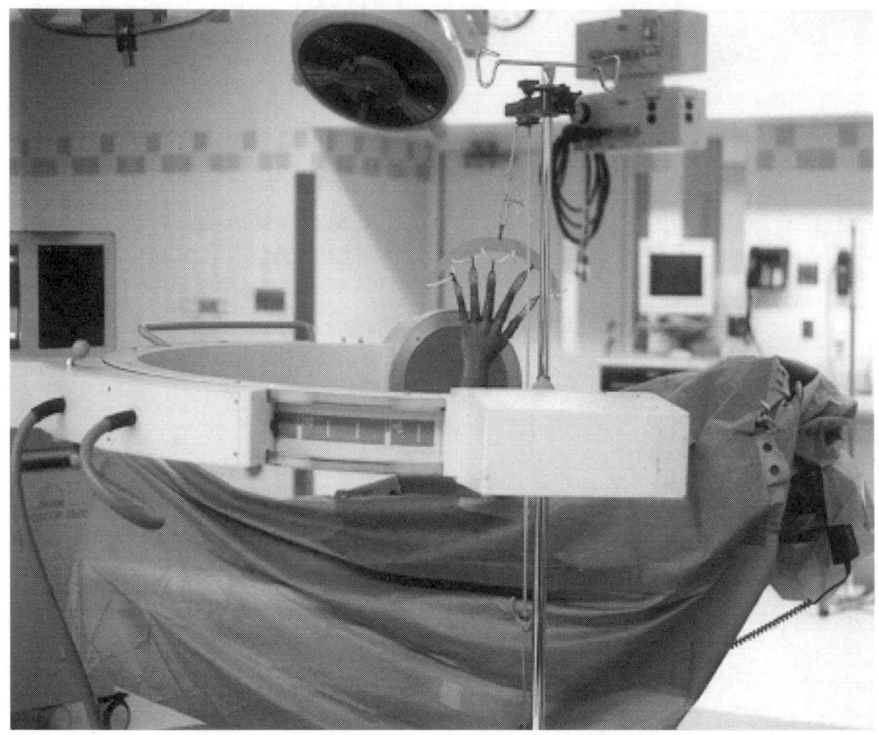

Figure 28.1 *C-arm in position of ap view.*

PATIENT POSITION: Patient will be supine with affected fingers in trap traction, arm skyward and elbow bent.

C-ARM POSITION: C-arm will enter perpendicular or at a 45 degree angle to patient. C-arm will be tilted until the image intensifier is parallel to floor.

Notes: When rotating c-arm ensure patient is properly positioned to allow you to safely move the image intensifier.

Allow for working space of surgeon.

Position image intensifier close to wrist to create a larger field of view.

Drape both ends of c-arm with snap cover drape to allow maximum movement.

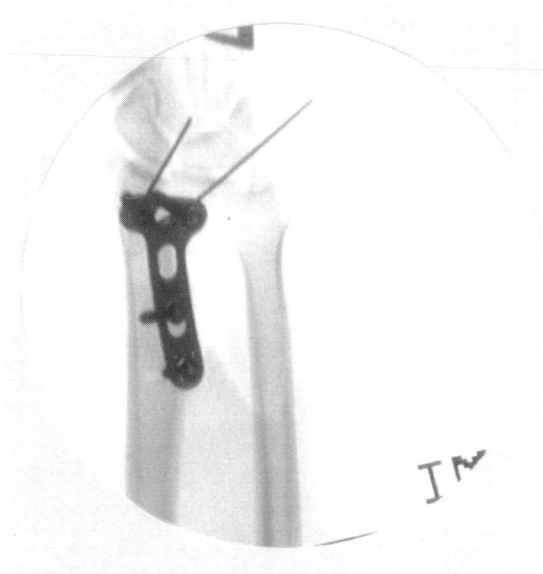

Figure 28.2 *X-ray image of wrist with pins inserted.*

29. WRIST/FINGER PINNING
(USING FINGERTRAPS LATERAL POSITION)

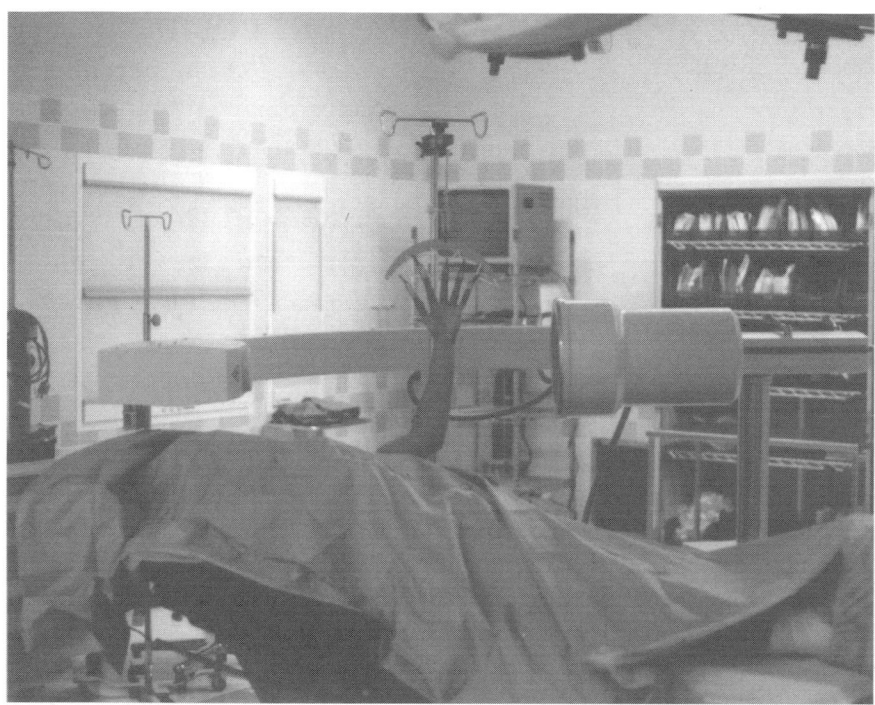

Figure 29.1 *C-arm in position of lateral view.*

PATIENT POSITION: Patient will be supine with affected fingers in trap traction arm skyward and elbow bent.

C-ARM POSITION: C-arm will enter perpendicular or at a 45 degree angle to patient. C-arm will be tilted until the image intensifier is parallel to floor. Rotate the C forward or backward until the true lateral is obtained.

Notes: When rotating c-arm, ensure that patient is properly positioned to allow you to safely move the image intensifier.

Allow for working space of surgeon.

Position image intensifier close to wrist to create a larger field of view.

Drape both ends of c-arm with snap cover drape to allow maximum movement.

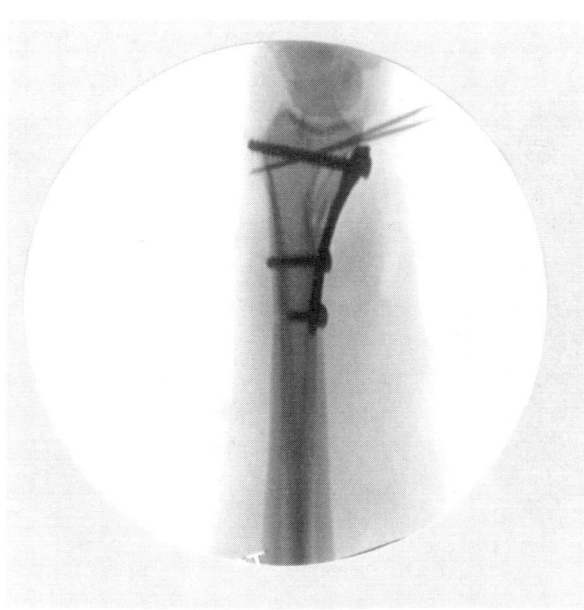

Figure 29.2 *X-ray image of wrist with pins inserted.*

30. FOOT/METATARSAL PINNING
(USING FINGER TRAPS AP POSITION)

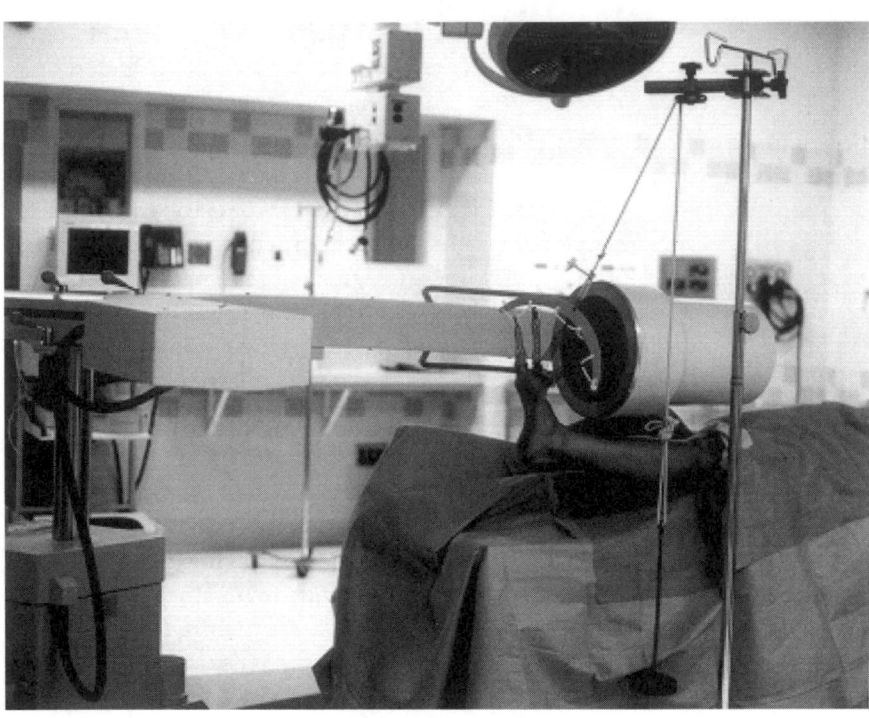

Figure 30.1 *C-arm in position of ap view.*

PATIENT POSITION:
Patient will be supine with affected toes in trap traction and leg raised skyward.

C-ARM POSITION: C-arm will enter with the C tilted to 90 degrees and image intensifier parallel to floor.

Notes: Ensure that the unaffected leg is safely positioned when lowering c-arm.

Position image intensifier close to foot to create a larger field of view.

C-arm may have to be rotated forward or backward to create true ap view.

Drape both ends of c-arm with snap cover drape to allow maximum movement.

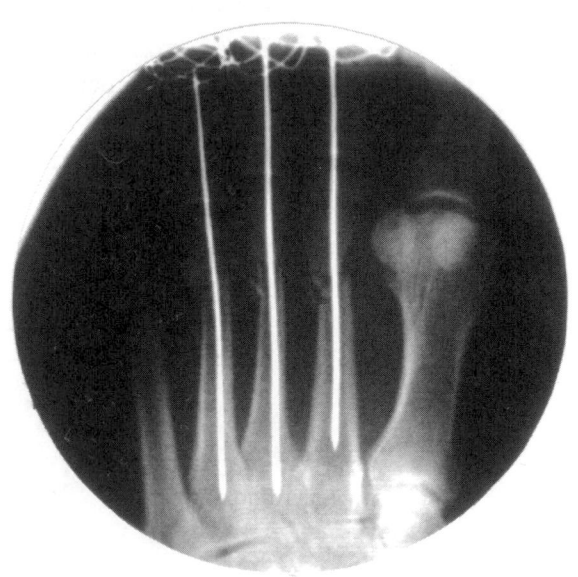

Figure 30.2 *X-ray image of metatarsal with pins inserted.*

31. FOOT/METATARSAL PINNING
(USING FINGERTRAPS LATERAL POSITION)

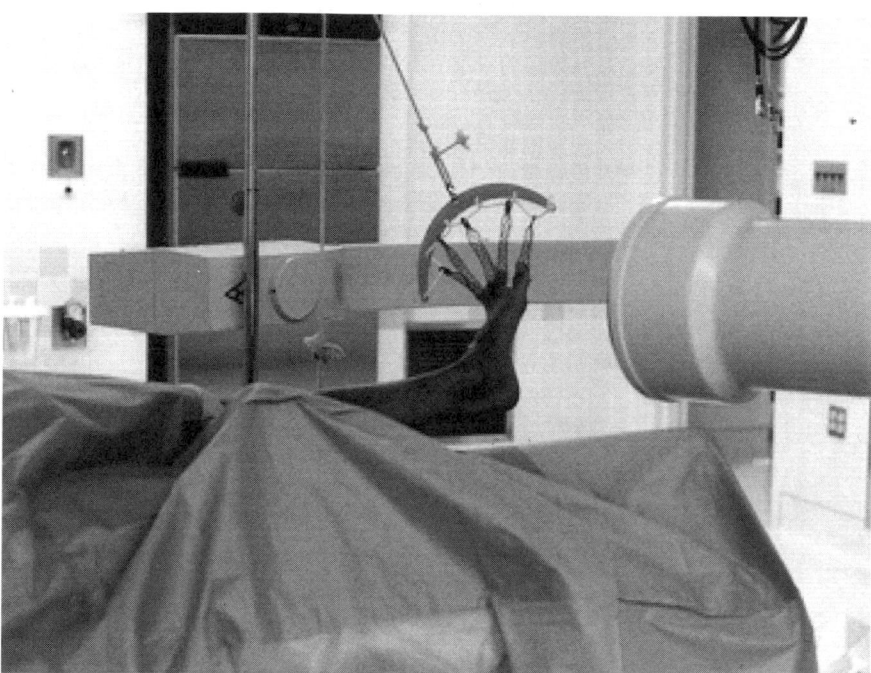

Figure 31.1 *C-arm in position of lateral view.*

PATIENT POSITION: Patient will be supine with affected toes in trap traction and leg raised skyward.

C-ARM POSITION: C-arm will enter with the C tilted to 90 degrees and image intensifier parallel to floor. Rotate the C forward or backward to obtain a true lateral view.

Notes: Ensure that the unaffected leg is safely positioned when lowering c-arm.

Position image intensifier close to foot to create a larger field of view.

Drape both ends of c-arm with snap cover drape to allow maximum movement.

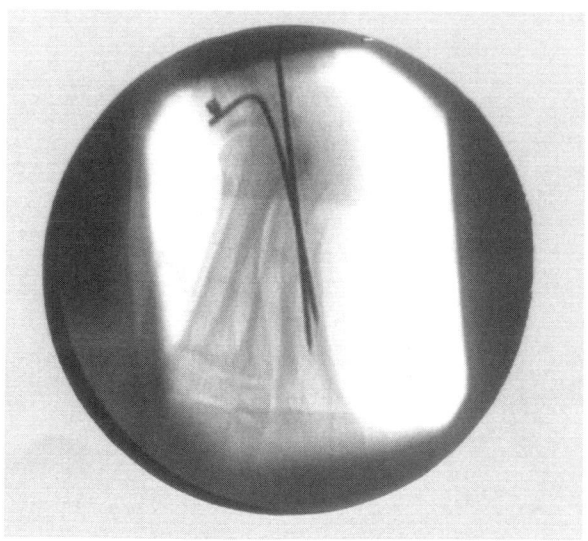

Figure 31.2 *X-ray image of metatarsal with pins inserted.*

32. CERVICAL ONE SPINAL FUSION
(AP POSITION)

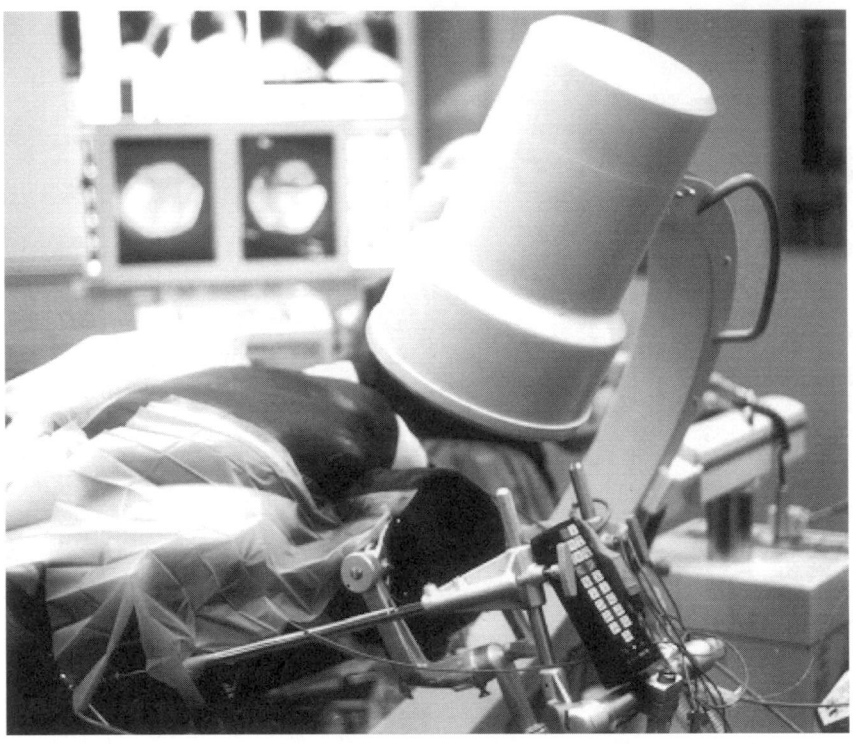

Figure 32.1 *C-arm in pa projection of cervical spine.*

PATIENT POSITION: Patient will be prone with head in harness and chin tilted downward.

C-ARM POSITION: C-arm will enter in ap projection, then angle caudal or cephalad to view C-1 cervical clearly.

Notes: Ensure area underneath is clear for movement of c-arm.

Be careful not to contribute to cervical instability by bumping head harness.

Collimate to eliminate burnout of cervical area.

To angle caudal with c-arm to view the body of cervical one is called Anderson's View.

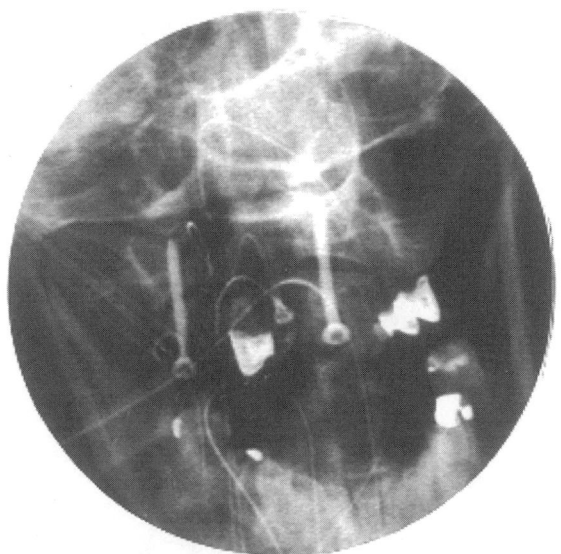

Figure 32.2 *C-arm image of cervical spine with screws inserted.*

33. CERVICAL ONE SPINAL FUSION
(LATERAL POSITION)

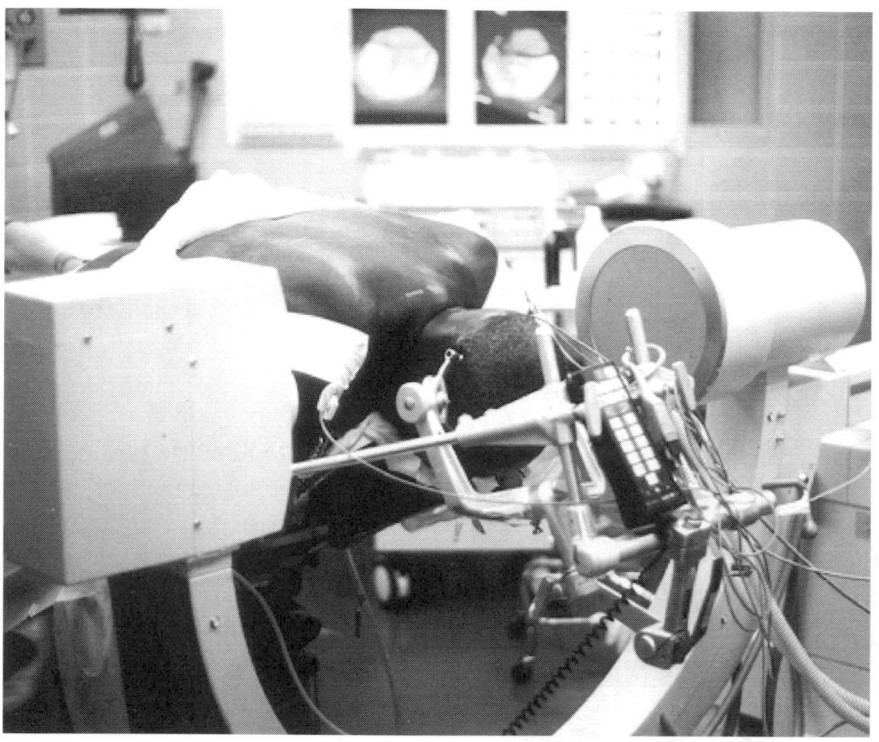

Figure 33.1 *C-arm in lateral projection of cervical spine.*

PATIENT POSITION:
Patient will be prone with head in harness and chin tilted downward.

C-ARM POSITION: C-arm will enter in ap projection, then rotate underneath table to lateral position.

Notes: Be careful not to bump head instrumentation when moving c-arm.

Wigwag c-arm to create true lateral view.

Pins will protrude from spine a distance that will cause concern of possible puncture of c-arm drape.

Be sure not to dislodge lines or cables underneath table.

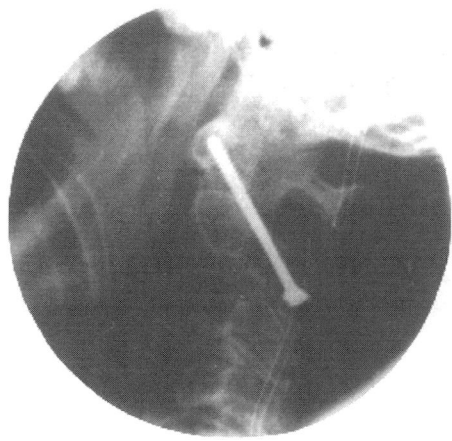

Figure 33.2 *C-arm image of cervical spine with screws inserted.*

34. INTERBODY FUSION DEVICE
(AP POSITION)

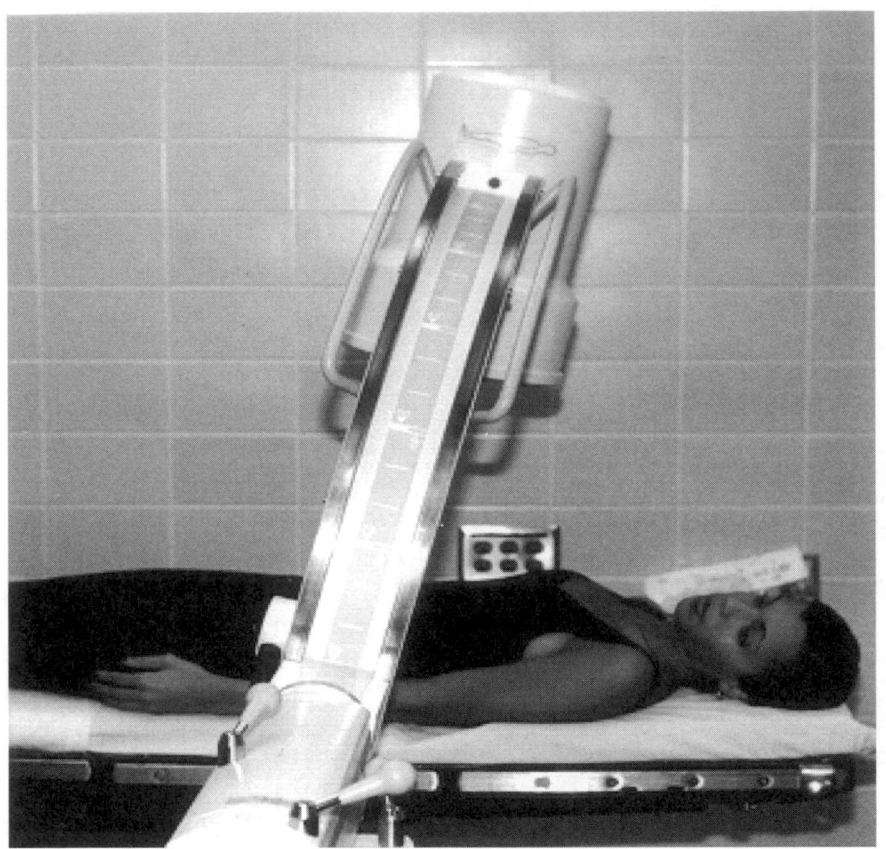

Figure 34.1 *C-arm in ap projection of spine.*

PATIENT POSITION: Patient will be in the supine position with abdomen area on radiolucent table. A back roll may be utilized to extend the spine

C-ARM POSITION: C-arm will enter the patient in the ap projection. C-arm will be rotated underneath table to acquire the lateral view.

Notes: During ap projection ensure not to bump or dislodge laproscopic instrumentation.

The physician may require Furgenson view.
Angle c-arm caudal 10 to 25 degrees to align cage in circular projection.

In the lateral view it may be necessary to angle c-arm caudal or cephalad depending on the stenosis.

Ensure area underneath table is clear of lines during movement to lateral position.

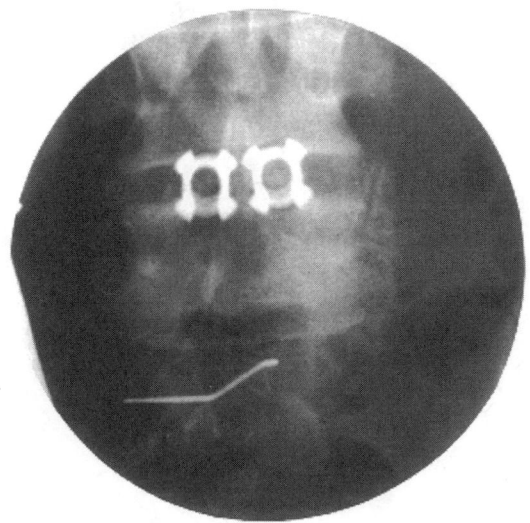

Figure 34.2 *C-arm image of ap spine with interbody fusion device in place.*

35. INTERBODY FUSION DEVICE
(LATERAL POSITION)

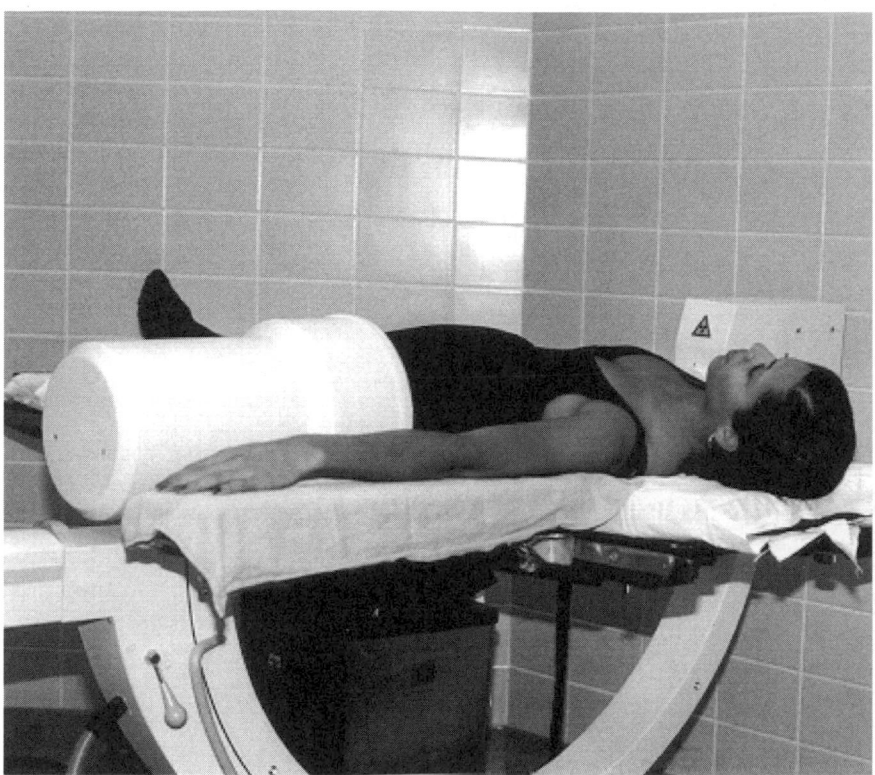

Figure 35.1 *C-arm in lateral projection of spine.*

PATIENT POSITION: Patient will be in the supine position with abdomen area on radiolucent table. A back roll may be utilized to extend the spine.

C-ARM POSITION: Rotate c-arm underneath table to acquire the lateral view.

Notes: During lateral view it may be necessary to angle c-arm caudal or cephalad depending on the stenosis. This view is called the Laurnen's Angle.

Ensure area underneath table is clear of lines during movement to lateral position.

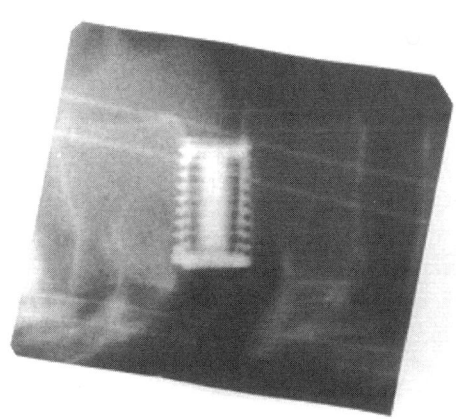

Figure 35.2 *X-ray image of lateral spine with interbody fusion device in place.*

36. POSTERIOR LATERAL FUSION WITH PLATES OR RODS
(PA POSITION)

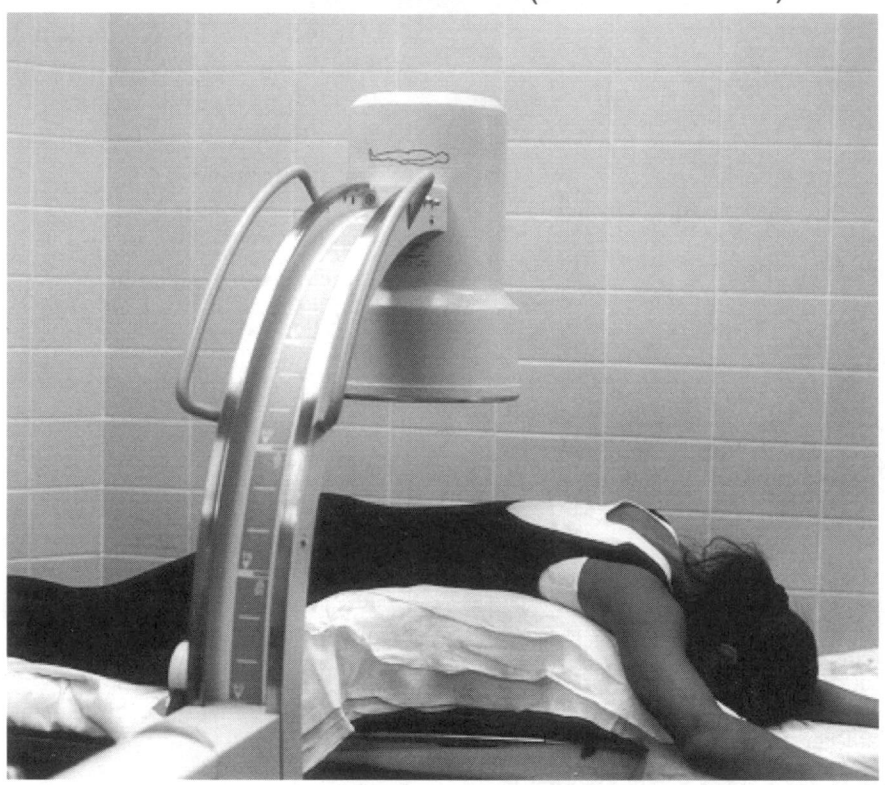

PATIENT POSITION: Patient will be prone and flexed in the spinal area.

C-ARM POSITION: C-arm will be positioned over spinal area of fusion.

Notes: It may be necessary to rotate c-arm over or backward to obtain true pa view of spine.

During pa view, patients with scoliosis may require tilting of c-arm to open disc space.

Procedure must be performed on a radiolucent table to be able to obtain this view.

Figure 36.1 *C-arm in pa projection of spine.*

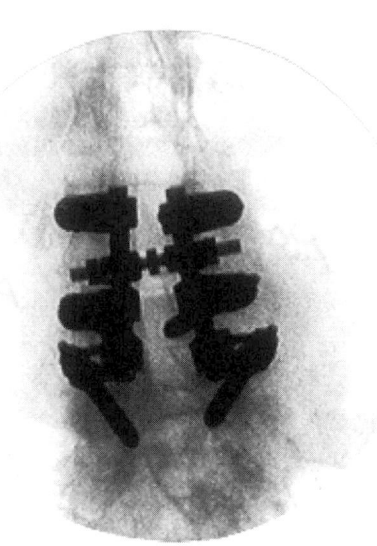

Figure 36.2 *C-arm image of pa spine with instrumentation.*

37. POSTERIOR LATERAL FUSION WITH PLATES OR RODS
(LATERAL POSITION)

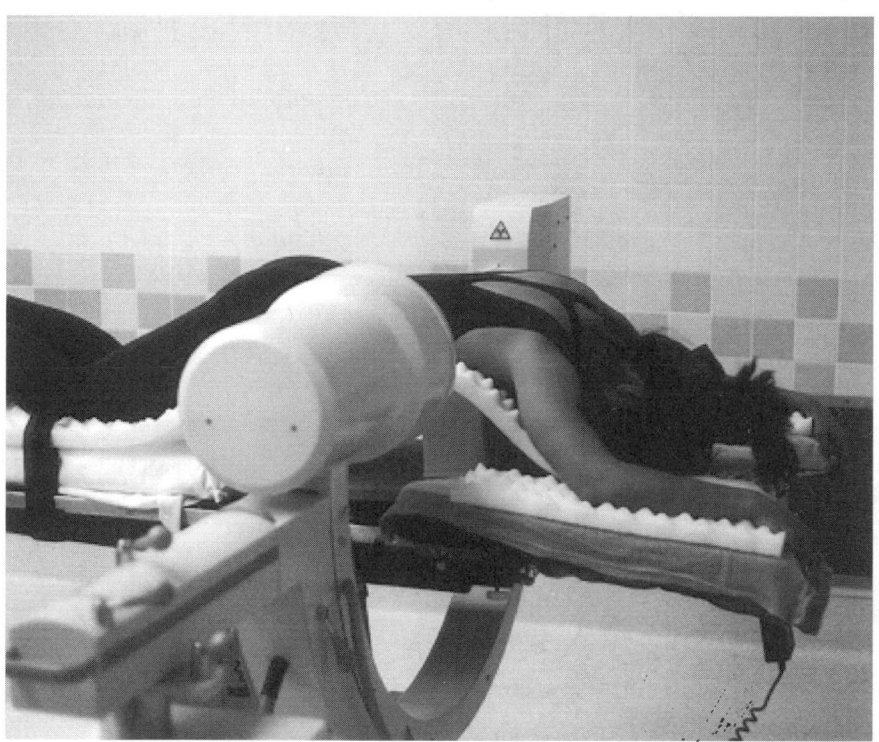

Figure 37.1 *C-arm in lateral projection of spine.*

PATIENT POSITION: Patient will be prone and flexed in the spinal area.

C-ARM POSITION: C-arm will be rotated underneath table to a lateral projection.

Notes: When performing a lateral view on a patient with scoliosis, it may be necessary to wig-wag the c-arm to align the spine. This view is called Laurnen's Angle.

It may be necessary to angle caudal or cephaliad to obtain true lateral of spine.

During lateral view, patients with scoliosis may require tilting of c-arm to open disc space.

A spine program on the c-arm best illustrates this view.

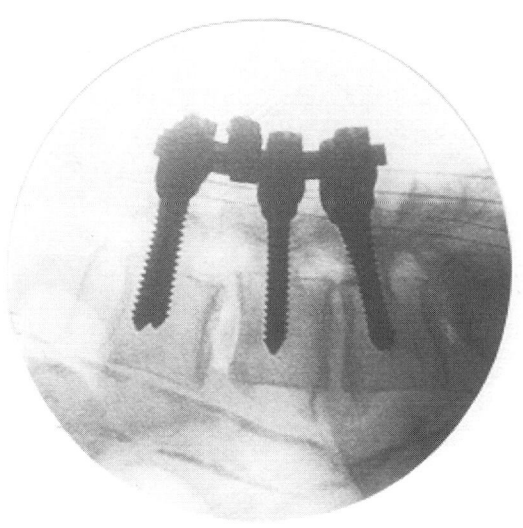

Figure 37.2 *C-arm image of lateral spine with fusion in place.*

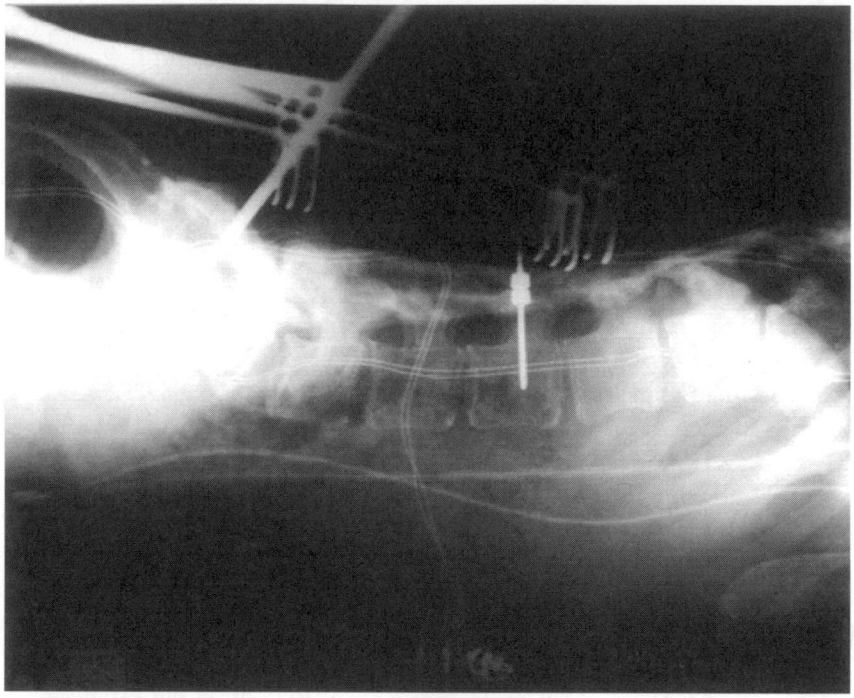

Figure 37.3 *When creating a fluoroscopic imaging of the spine during implantations, scatter radiation can affect the quality of the image. A soft technique with the c-arm may best visualize these areas. Image shown without using soft technique.*

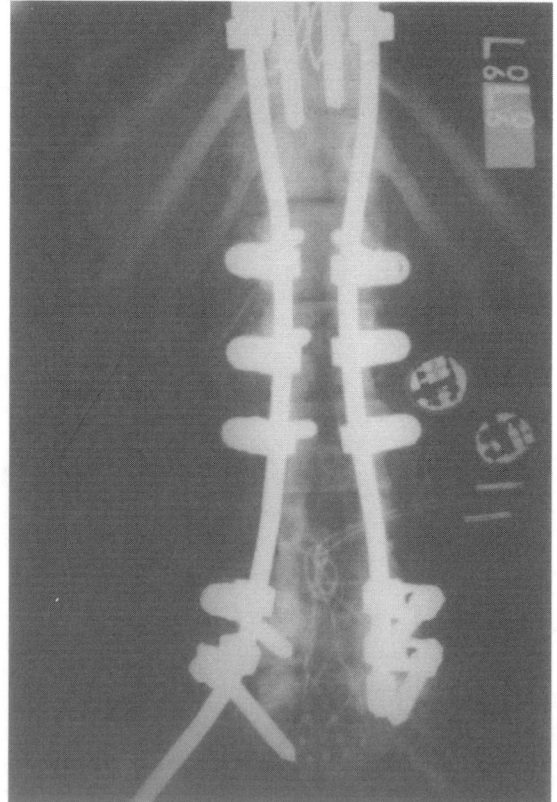

Figure 37.4 *The pa spine, using a soft technique on the c-arm.*

38. DEEP BRAIN STIMULATOR
(AP VIEW)

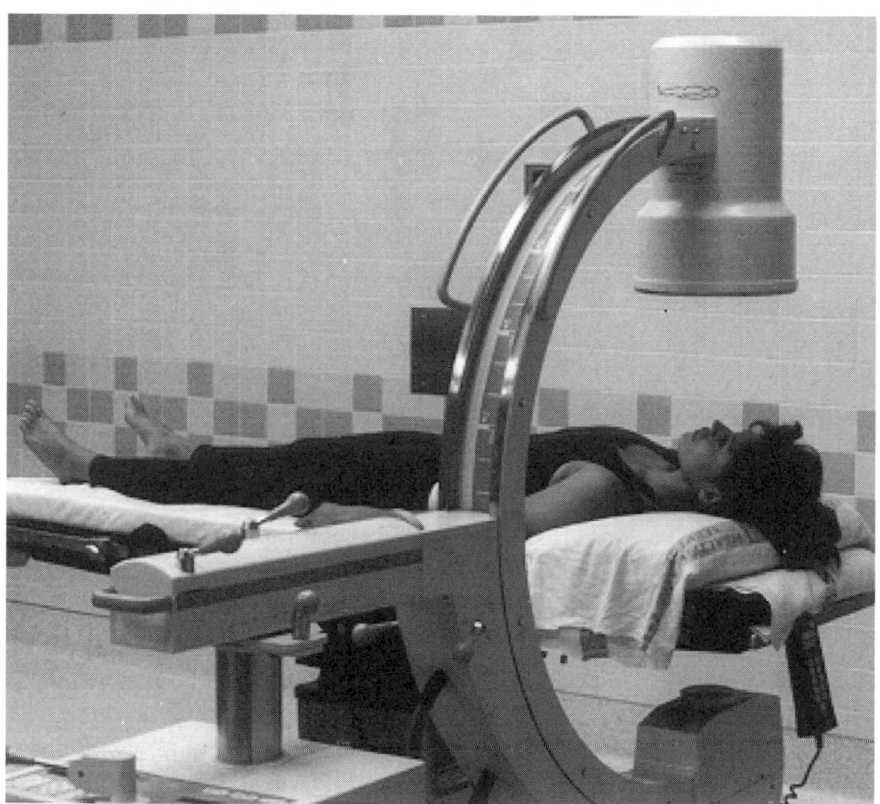

PATIENT POSITION: Patient will be supine and flexed at the hips in a semi-sitting position.

C-ARM POSITION: C-arm will enter perpendicular to the patient and on line with the skull.

Notes: Ensure not to bump head brace when positioning for the view of the ap skull.

C-arm may have to be tilted to create a true ap of the skull.

C-arm may have to be rotated to view stimulator in position of the brain.

Figure 38.1 *C-arm in projection of ap skull.*

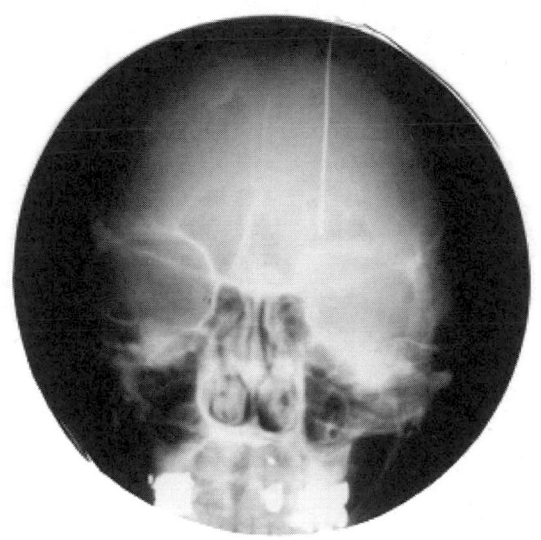

Figure 38.2 *X-ray image of lateral skull with stimulator inserted.*

39. DEEP BRAIN STIMULATOR

(LATERAL VIEW)

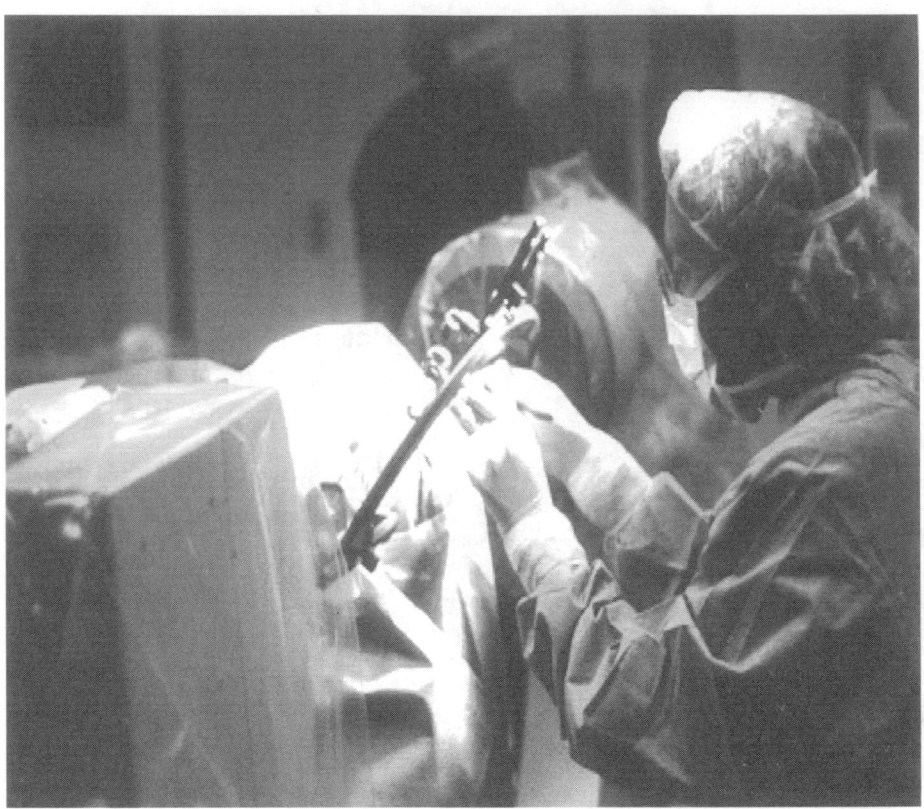

Figure 39.1 *C-arm in projection of lateral skull.*

PATIENT POSITION:
Patient will be supine with
the neck and upper torso
flexed and in the semi-sitting
position.

C-ARM POSITION: C-arm
will enter perpendicular to the
patient and on line with the
skull. Rotate c-arm underneath table to obtain the
lateral view.

Notes: Be careful not to
bump headbrace when
rotating to the lateral view. C-
arm might have to be tilted in
the lateral position to avoid
brace underneath table. C-
arm might need to enter from
the end of the table if the
brace does not allow for
underneath rotation.

Manipulate c-arm to center
and align target crosshairs on
headbrace.

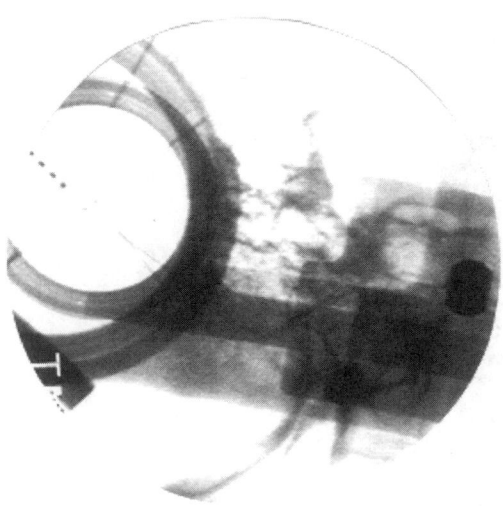

Figure 39.2 *X-ray image of lateral skull with stimulator inserted.*

40. OMAYA RESERVOIR PLACEMENT

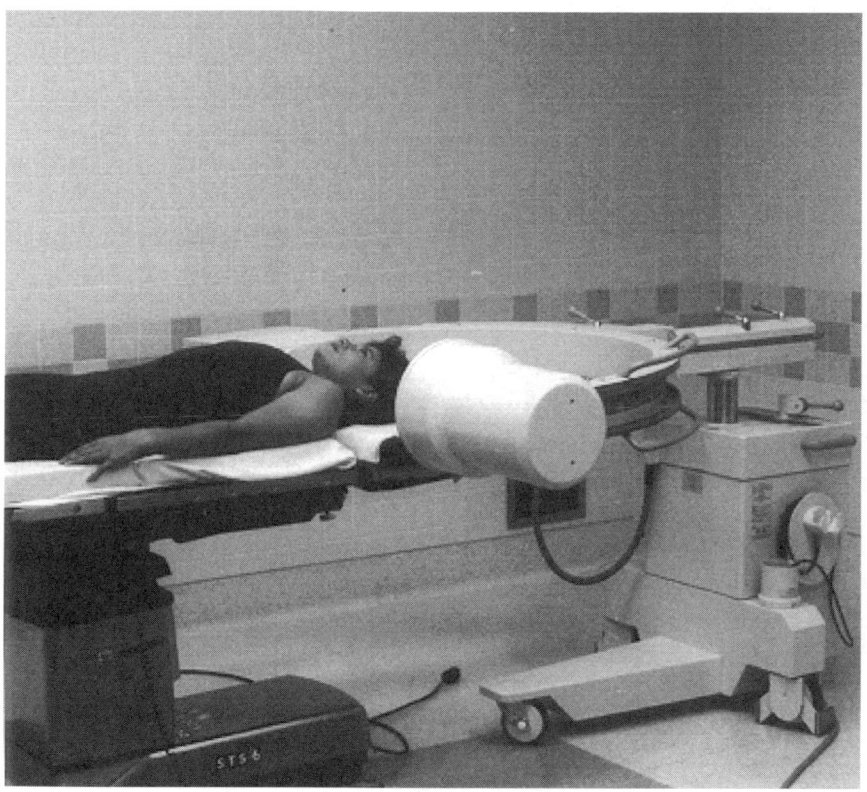

Figure 40.1 *C-arm in lateral projection of skull.*

PATIENT POSITION: Patient will be supine. Head may be slightly tilted to the right or left.

C-ARM POSITION: C-arm will enter in the ap projection of skull then rotated underneath to the lateral view if necessary.

Notes: Move image intensifier close to skull to create a larger field of view.

Drape c-arm on both ends with banded type sterile drape.

Contrast may be injected to enhance position.

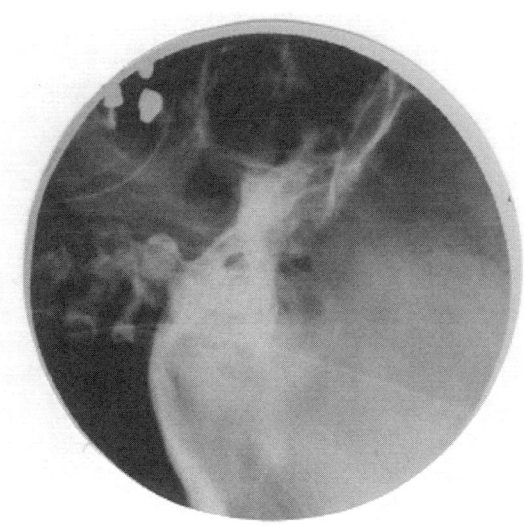

Figure 40.2 *X-ray image of lateral skull.*

41. TRANSPHENOID RESECTION OF PITUITARY TUMOR

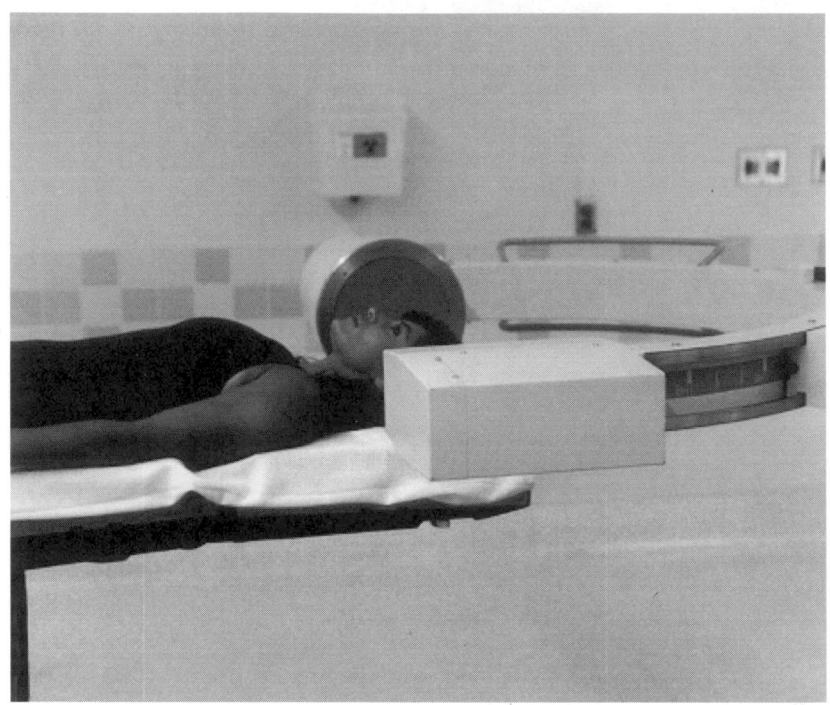

PATIENT POSITION: Patient will be supine and in a slight sitting position.

C-ARM POSITION: C-arm will enter at patient's head with the "C" tilted parallel to surface projecting a true lateral image of skull.

Notes: C-arm may have to be rotated in a circular motion or tilted to create a true lateral of the skull. The pituitary should be centered on the screen, with the orbits super imposed. This is called the Raisis View.

Figure 41.1 *C-arm in lateral projection of skull.*

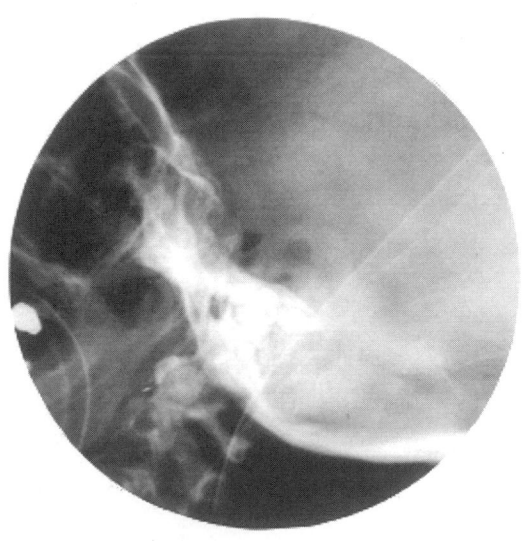

Figure 41.2 *C-arm image of lateral skull.*

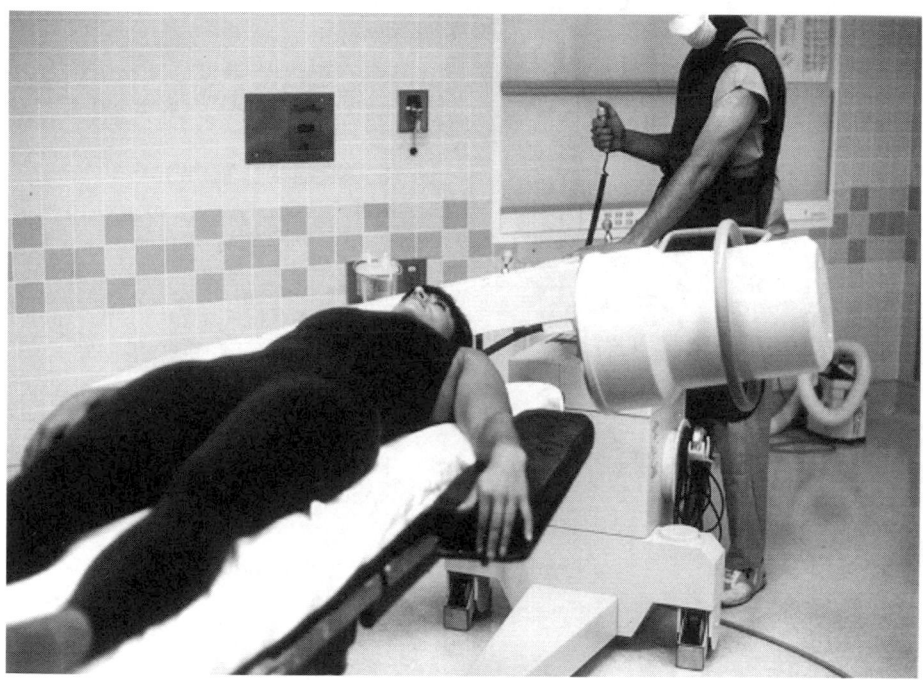

Figure 41.3. *To align the pituitary area the c-arm may have to be tilted to overlay these areas.*

42. RADIO FREQUENCY RHIZOTOMY
(AP POSITION)

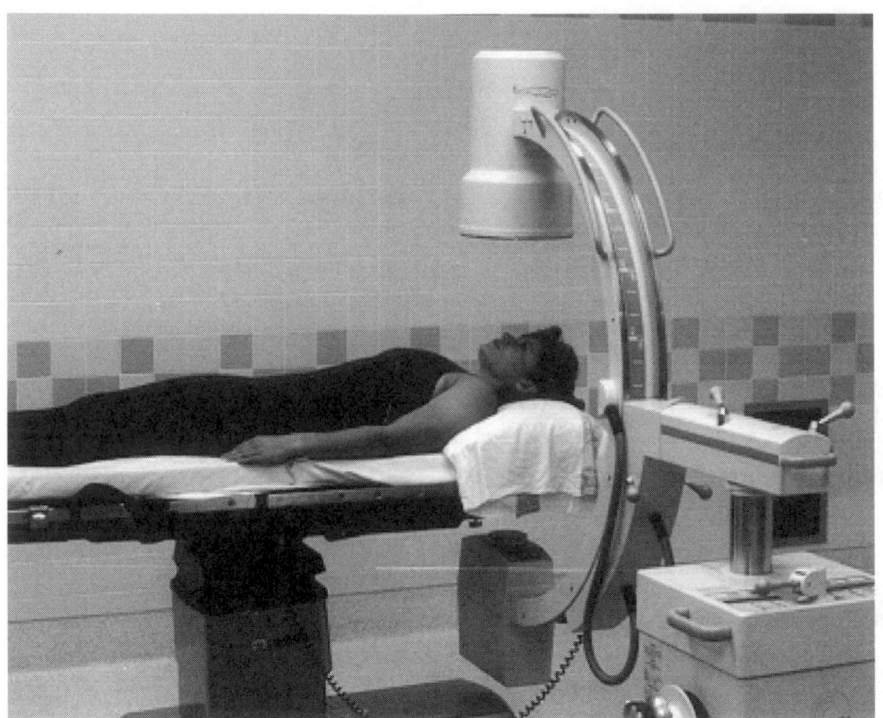

Figure 42.1 *C-arm in ap position of skull.*

PATIENT POSITION:
Patient will be supine on operating table with shoulders slightly elevated to assist in obtaining SMV if needed.

C-ARM POSITION: C-arm will be positioned over patient's skull.

Notes: The technologist may be asked to display a SMV projection. C-arm fluoroscopy is used while surgeon inserts probes into the trigeminal space.

Images should adequately demonstrate the area of interest, particularly anatomy of the sella turcica.

Patient will be sedated, but not asleep for procedure.

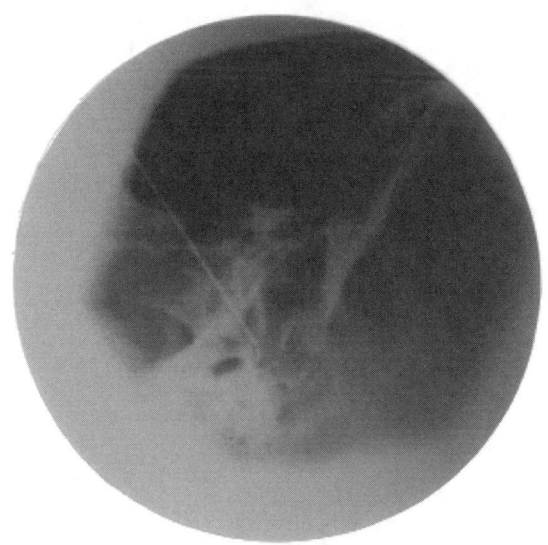

Figure 42.2 *C-arm image of ap skull with probe in place.*

43. RADIO FREQUENCY RHIZOTOMY
(LATERAL POSITION)

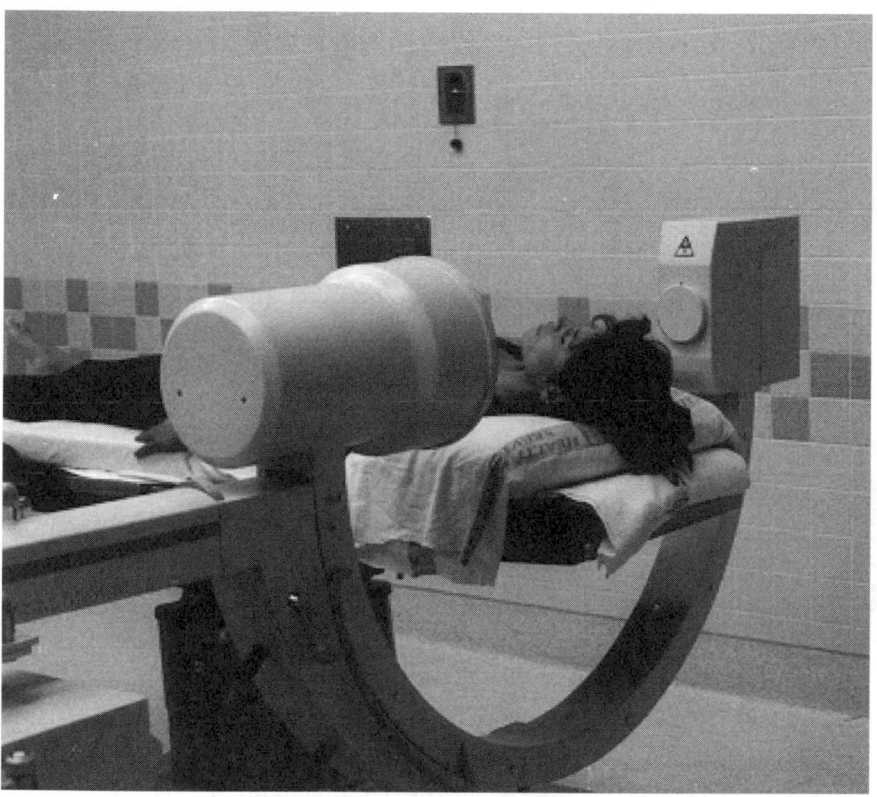

Figure 43.1 *C-arm in lateral position of skull.*

PATIENT POSITION: Patient will be supine on operating table with shoulders slightly elevated to assist in obtaining SMV if needed.

C-ARM POSITION: C-arm will be rotated underneath table with manipulation to create true lateral view.

Notes: The technologist may be asked to display an SMV projection.

Ensure area underneath is clear to allow movement of the C-arm.

C-arm may have to be manipulated to obtain a true lateral view.

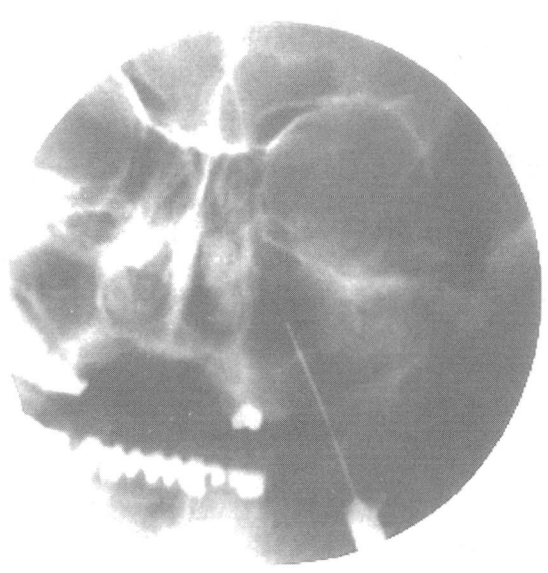

Figure 43.2 *C-arm image of lateral skull with probe in place.*

44. SHUNT PLACEMENT/ SHUNT REVISIONS

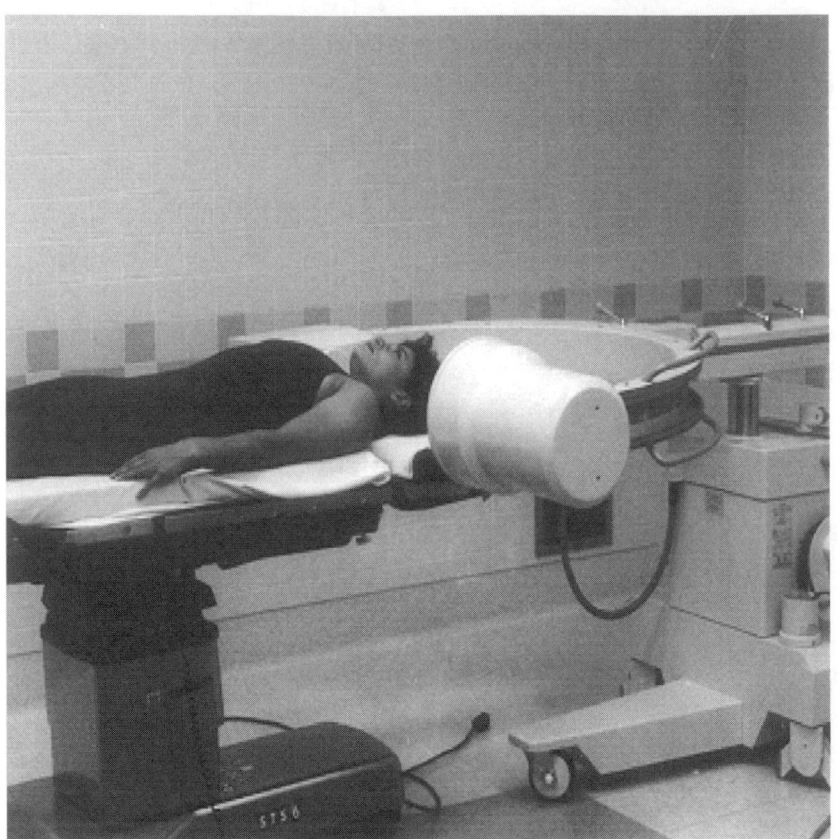

Figure 44.1 C-arm in position of lateral skull.

PATIENT POSITION: Patient will be supine with arm along the side. Patient's head will be straight up or with the head turned to the right or left depending on shunt site.

C-ARM POSITION: C-arm will enter over patient's skull projected in the ap position. If a lateral view is desired, rotate c-arm forward or backward to obtain lateral view.

Notes: It is important that a true lateral of the skull can be obtained.

Ensure that table is sufficient to view chest area.

Move image intensifier closer to skull for a larger field of view. Keep in mind working space for surgeon.

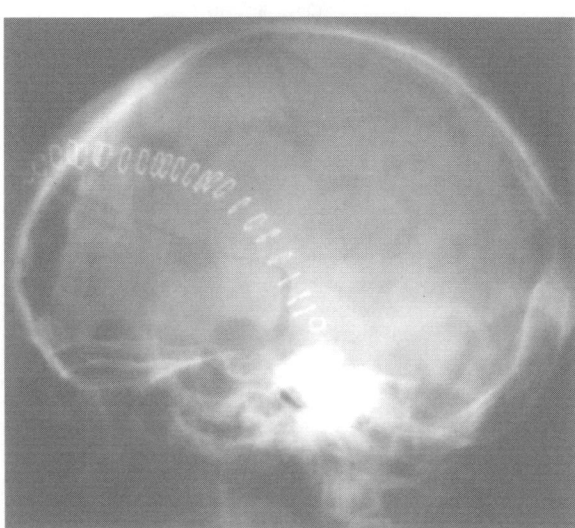

Figure 44.2 C-arm image of lateral skull.

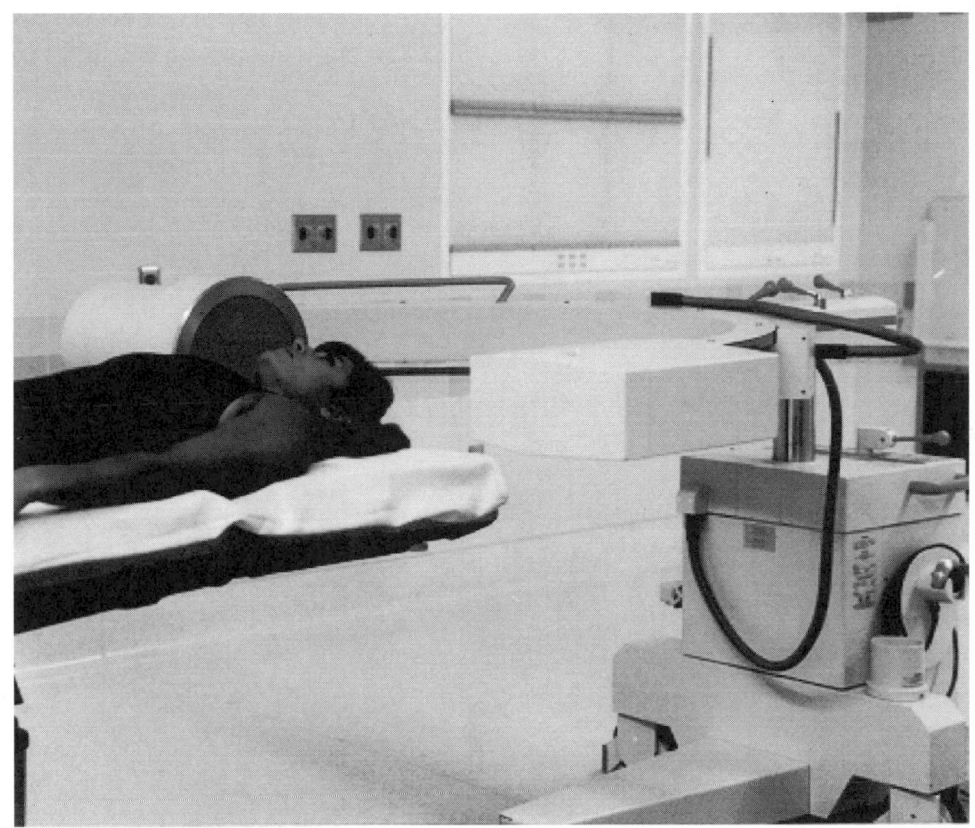

Figure 44.3 *During imaging of the skull, move the image intensifier close to the skull to promote a larger field of view.*

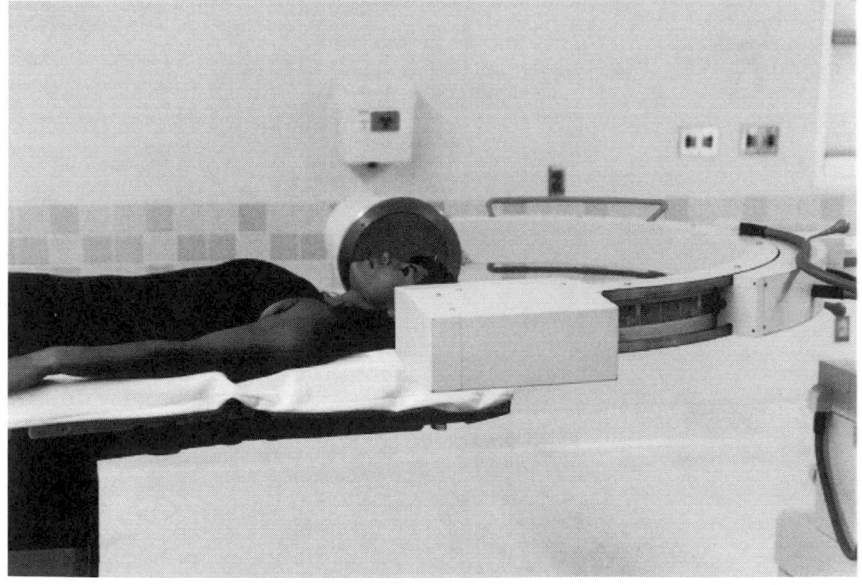

Figure 44.4 *During skull procedures tilt the c-arm to horizontal. With the ability to rotate around for alignment this position of the c-arm will allow for better imaging.*

45. EPIDURAL CATHETER INSERTION
(AP POSITION)

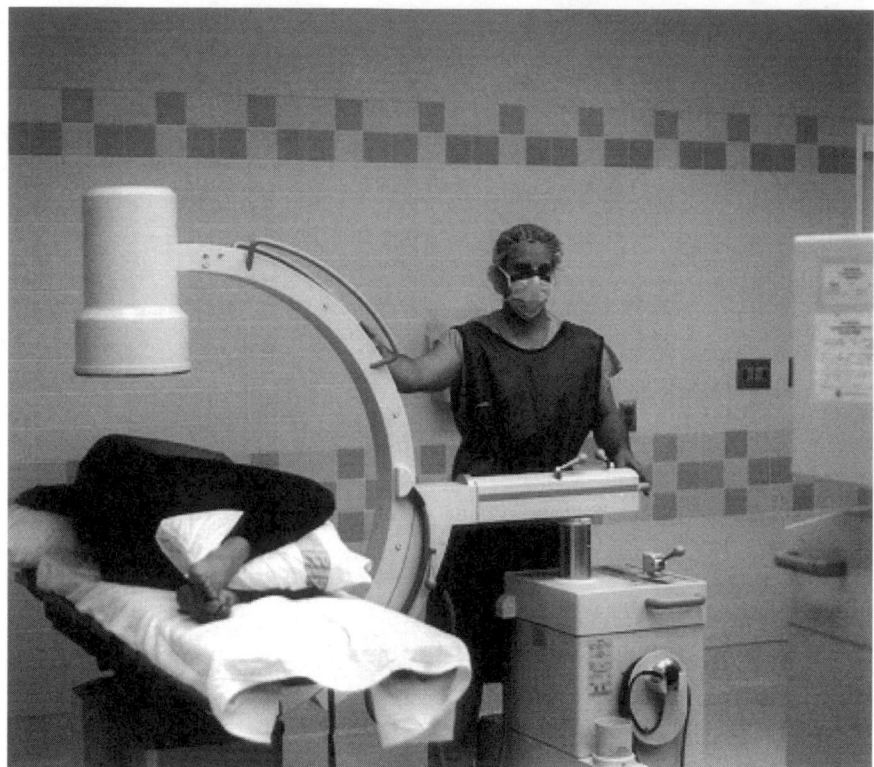

PATIENT POSITION: Patient will be in the lateral position with either right or left side down.

C-ARM POSITION: C-arm enters facing the patient then rotates underneath table to the ap projection.

Notes: Doctor will work to the posterior of patient.

Ensure area underneath table is clear for movement.

It may be necessary to wig-wag the c-arm to align disc space.

Figure 45.1 C-arm in ap projection of spine.

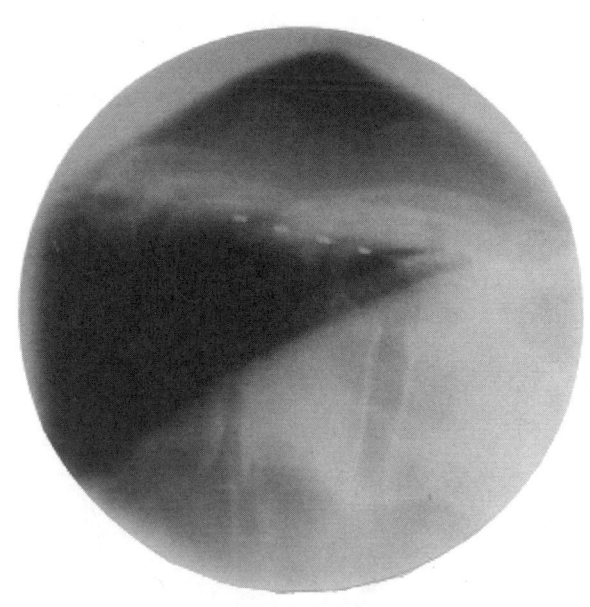

Figure 45.2 C-arm image of ap spine with catheter inserted.

46. EPIDURAL CATHETER INSERTION
(LATERAL POSITION)

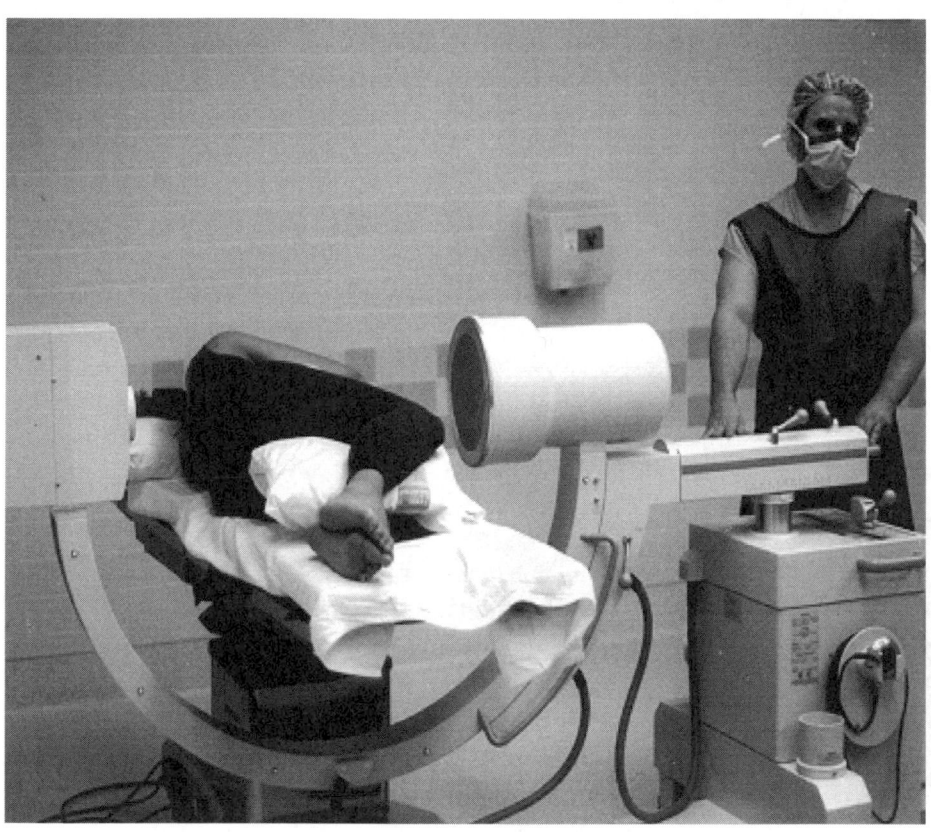

Figure 46.1 *C-arm in lateral projection of spine.*

PATIENT POSITION: Patient will be in the lateral position with either right or left side down.

C-ARM POSITION: C-arm enters facing the patient.

Notes: Doctor will work to the posterior of patient.

Ensure that a visibility of surgical area can be obtained.

Ap view may be obtained by rotating the c-arm underneath table to a cross table projection.

If patient has scoliosis it may be necessary to tilt c-arm cephalic or caudal to open disc space.

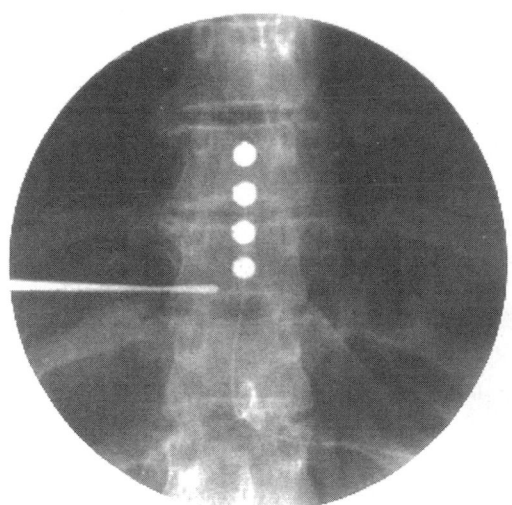

Figure 46.2 *C-arm image of lateral spine with catheter inserted.*

47. ALCOHOL CELIAC PLEXUS BLOCK
(AP POSITION)

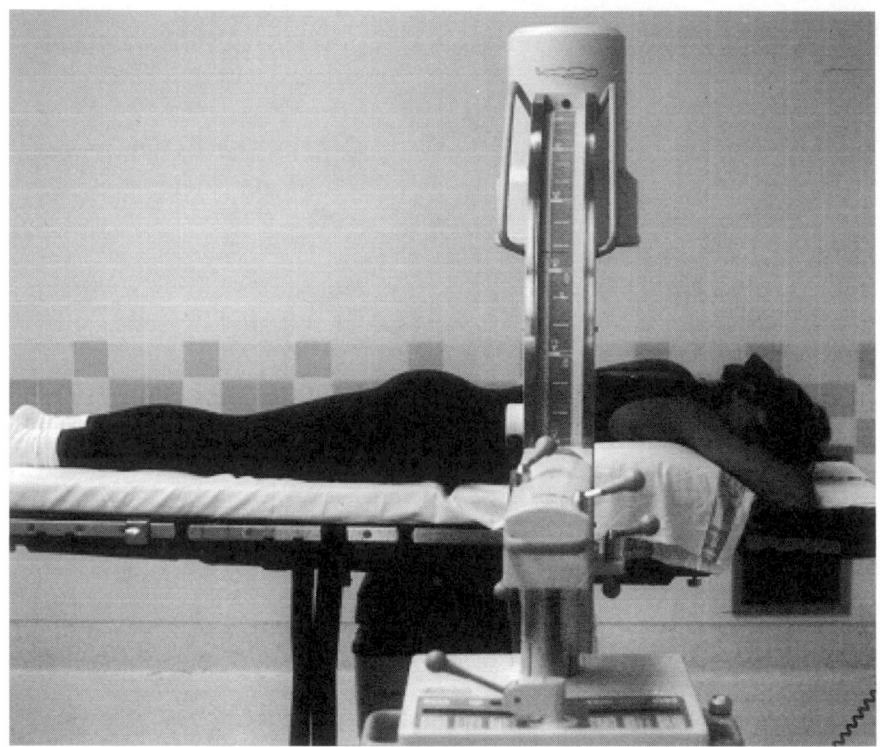

Figure 47.1 *C-arm in ap projection of spine.*

PATIENT POSITION: Patient will be prone with arms up near the shoulders.

C-ARM POSITION: C-arm will enter patient on either side in the ap projection. To obtain a lateral view rotate c-arm underneath table to the lateral projection.

Notes: Ensure not to dislodge needles when moving from the ap to lateral position.

Table may have to be raised when c-arm is in lateral position.

It may be necessary to angle c-arm to eliminate curvature of the spine.

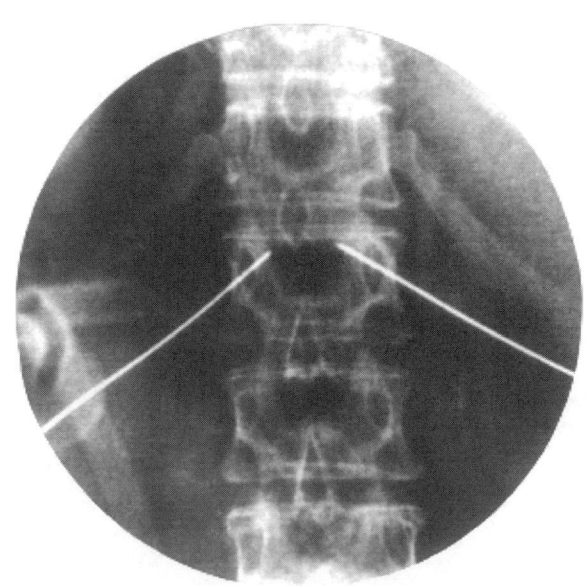

Figure 47.2 *C-arm image of ap spine with needles inserted.*

48. ALCOHOL CELIAC PLEXUS BLOCK
(LATERAL POSITION)

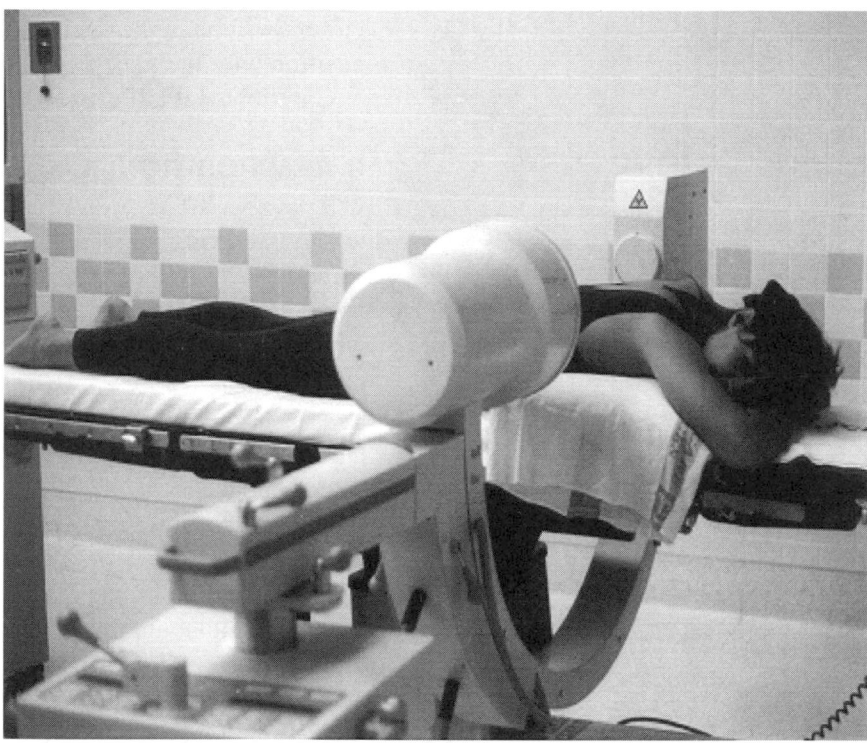

Figure 48.1 *C-arm in lateral projection of spine.*

PATIENT POSITION: Patient will be prone with arms at shoulder height.

C-ARM POSITION: C-arm will enter in the ap projection then rotate underneath table to the lateral projection.

Ensure not to dislodge needles when moving from the ap to lateral position.

Table should be clear and may have to be raised when c-arm is in lateral position.

Wig-wagging of the c-arm to eliminate lung markings and to align the disc space will give you Dupens' view.

Place image intensifier near the spine to create a larger field of view.

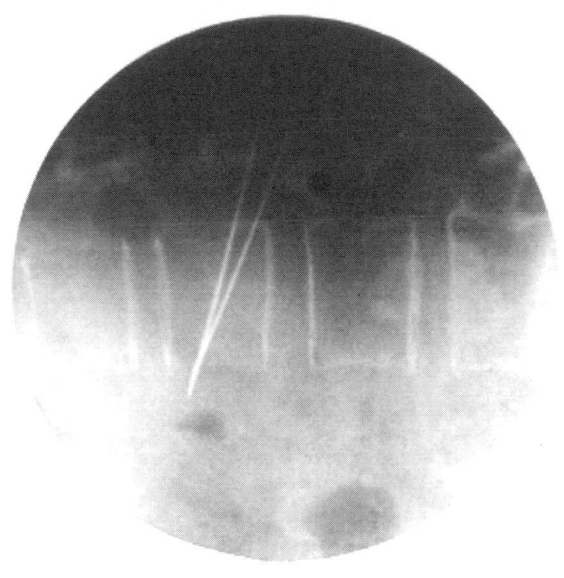

Figure 48.2 *C-arm image of lateral spine with needles inserted.*

49. LUMBAR DISCOGRAM
(PATIENT IN LATERAL POSITION)

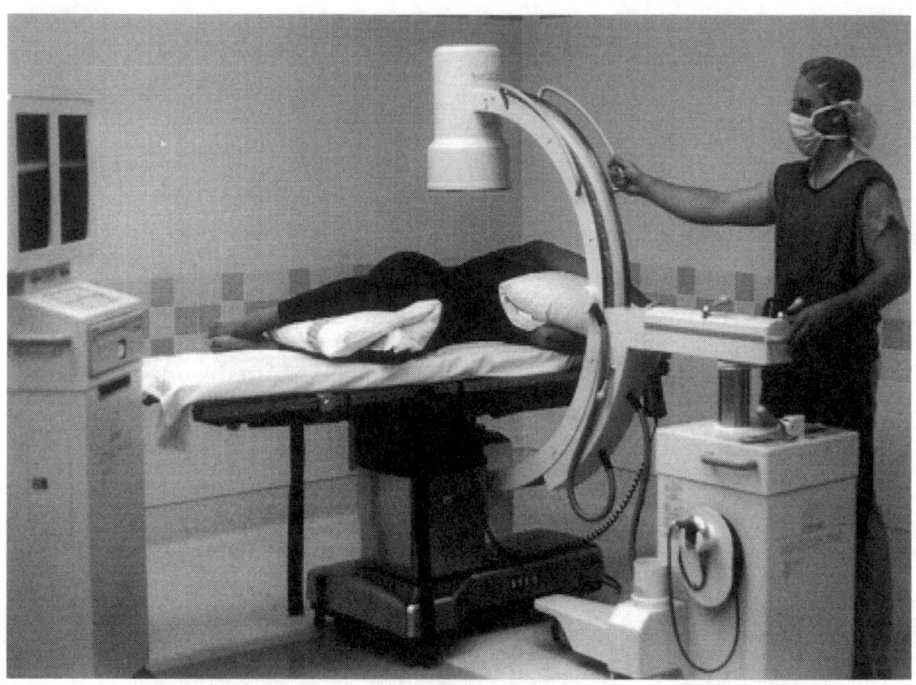

Figure 49.1 *C-arm in position for lateral lumbar spine.*

PATIENT POSITION:
Patient will be in the lateral position with the knee flexed on a radiolucent table.

C-ARM POSITION: C-arm will enter in the ap projection to show the view of lateral spine. C-arm will enter on opposite side of physician, who will be posterior to the patient.

Notes: C-arm may have to be tilted cephalad or caudal to open disc space.

A spine program on the c-arm will better illustrate this exam.

This exam may also be performed with the patient in the prone position.

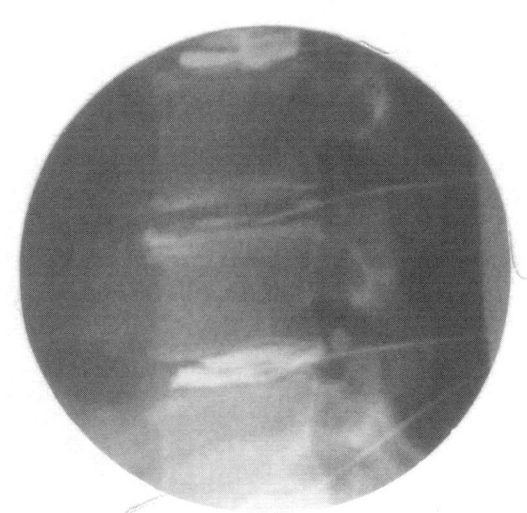

Figure 49.2 *C-arm image of lateral lumbar spine with contrast.*

50. LUMBAR FACET INJECTIONS
(PATIENT IN PRONE POSITION)

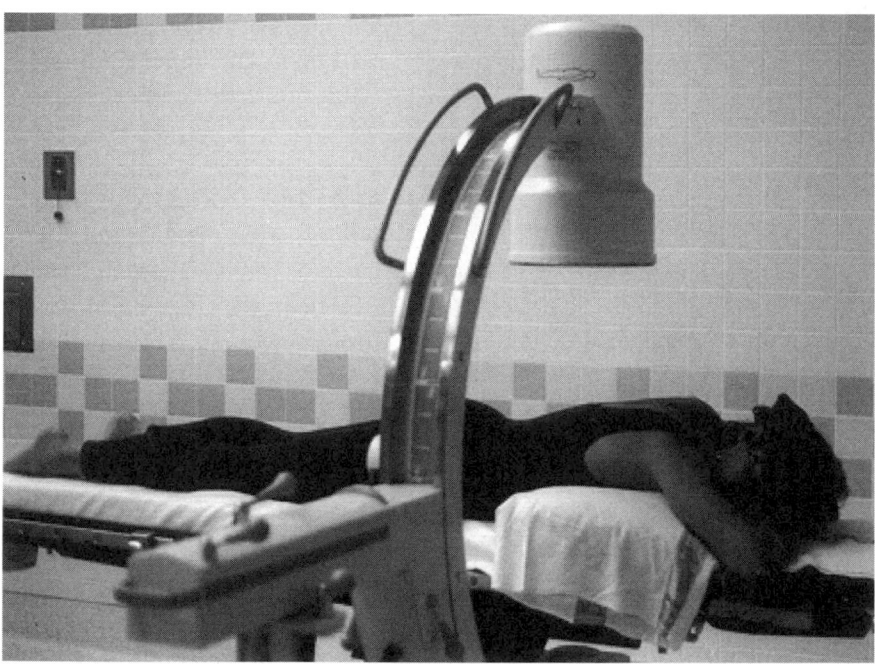

Figure 50.1 C-arm in pa projection of spine.

PATIENT POSITION: Patient will be prone on radiolucent table. Padding underneath abdomen may be used to flex the spine.

C-ARM POSITION: C-arm will enter perpendicular to the patient and in the p.a. projection of the spine on opposite side of physician.

Notes: C-arm may have to be rotated over or backwards to clearly expose needle in the facet.

A spine program on the c-arm will better illustrate this exam.

This exam may also be performed with the patient in the lateral position.

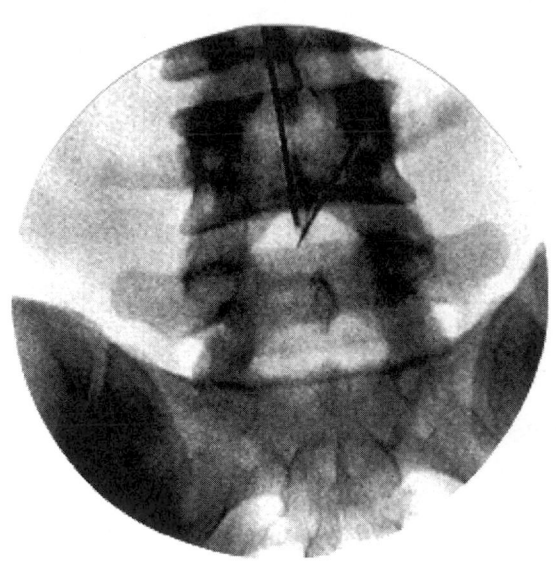

Figure 50.2 C-arm image pa lumbar spine.

51. IMPLANTABLE SPINAL MORPHINE PUMP

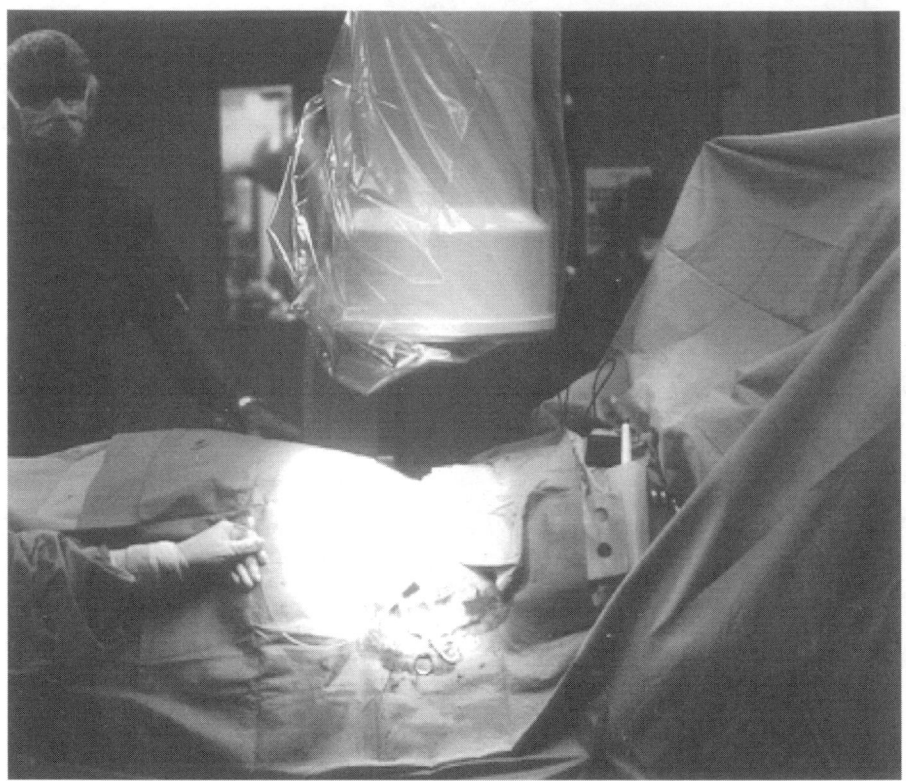

Figure 51.1 *C-arm in projection of lateral spine.*

PATIENT POSITION: Patient will be in the lateral position with either the right or left side down.

C-ARM POSITION: C-arm will enter perpendicular to and anterior to the patient. C-arm will be in the ap position projecting a lateral view of the spine.

Notes: Physician will be positioned posterior to the patient.

C-arm may have to be rotated over or backward to enhance imaging of the epidural space.

C-arm may have to be tilted left or right to align the disc space to show true indication of levels.

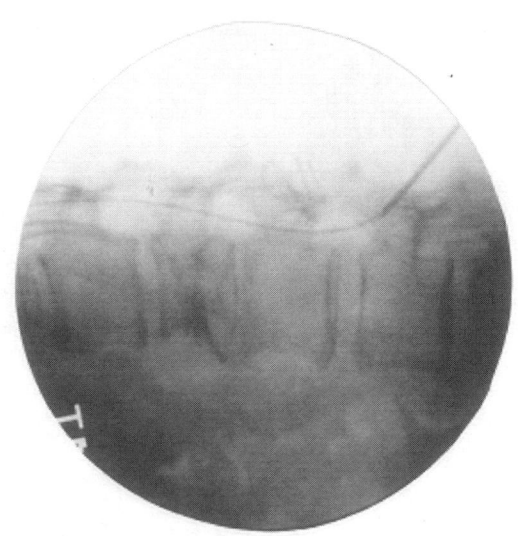

Figure 51.2 *X-ray image of lateral spine.*

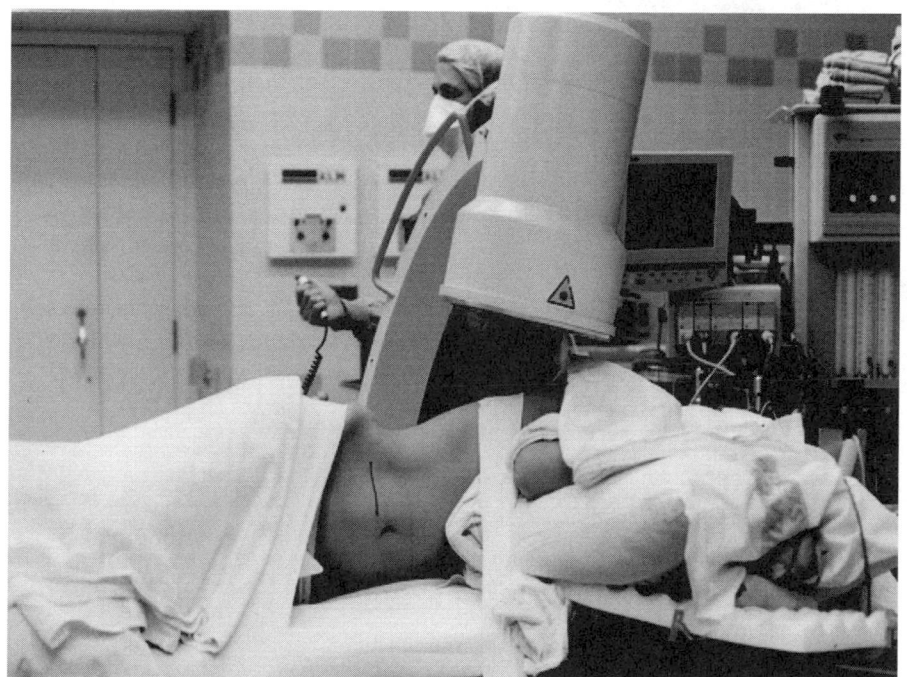

Figure 51.3 *The c-arm is tilted cephalad with the patient in the lateral position.*

Note that when performing pain management procedures with the patient in the lateral position, it may be necessary to tilt the c-arm cephalad or caudal if the patient has a scoliosis. Tilting the c-arm will open the disc space for better viewing.

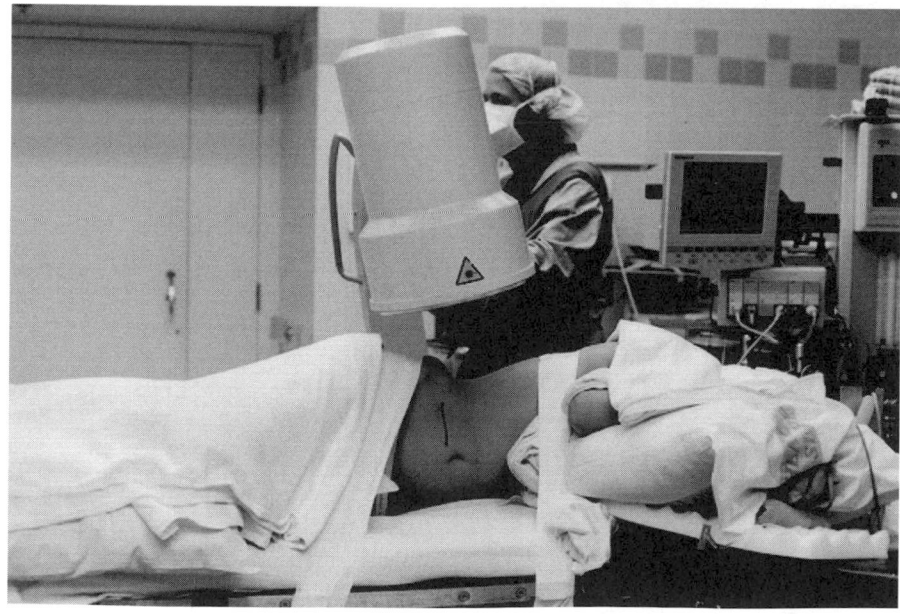

Figure 51.4 *The c-arm is tilted caudal with the patient in the lateral position.*

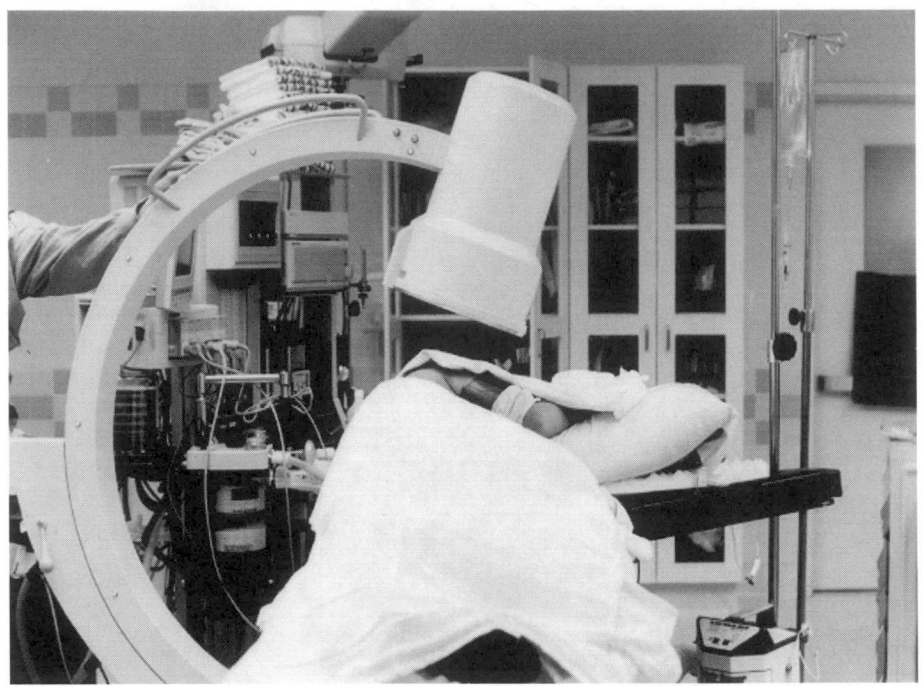

Figure 51.5 *The c-arm is rotated "over" with the patient in the lateral position.*

Note that when performing pain management examinations with the patient in the lateral position, it may be necessary to rotate the c-arm over or backward. This will align the spinous processes and promote a clear image of the dural space.

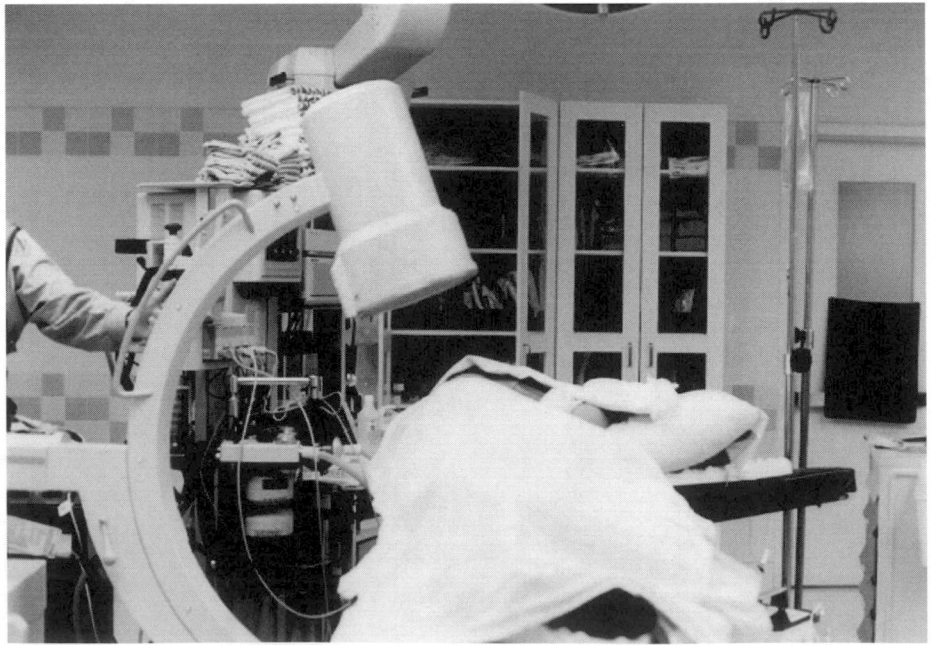

Figure 51.6 *Here the c-arm is rotated "back" with the patient in the lateral position.*

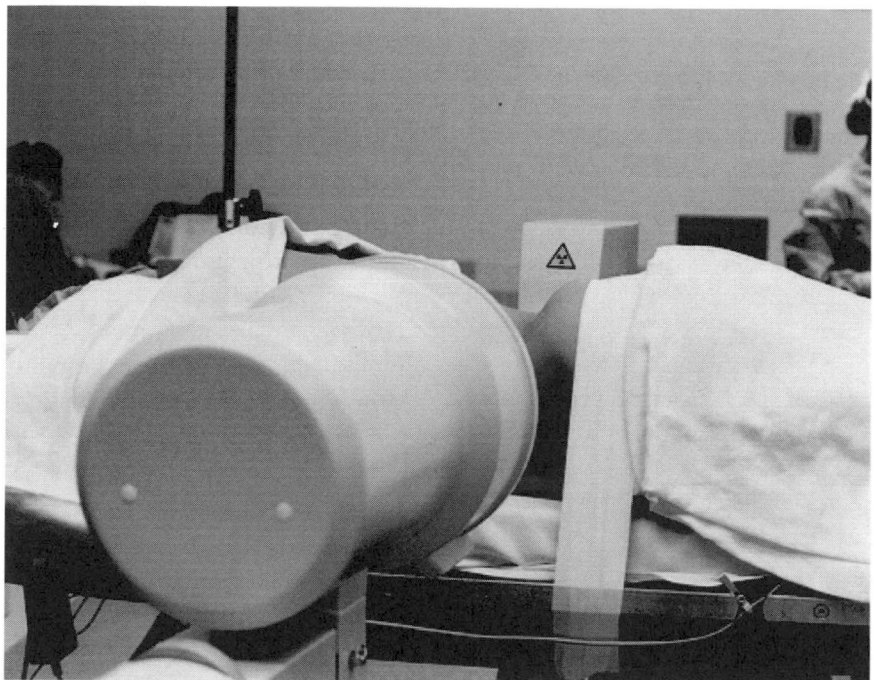

Figure 51.7 *Note that when performing cross table views during pain management procedures, the c-arm may have to be wig-wagged (angled) to view the disc space clearly.*

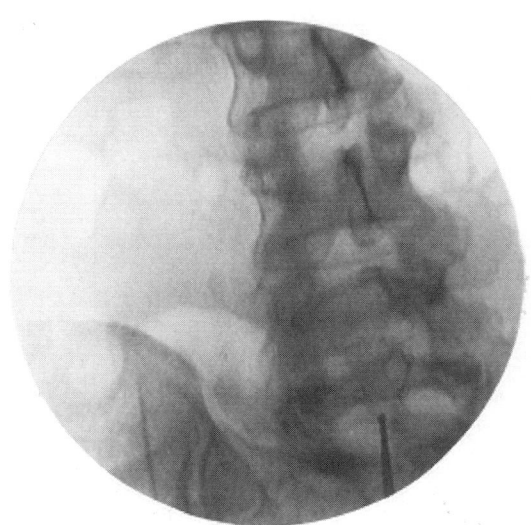

Figure 51.8 *Incorrect position of the spine.* **Note:** *The spinous process is not centered on the spinal body.*

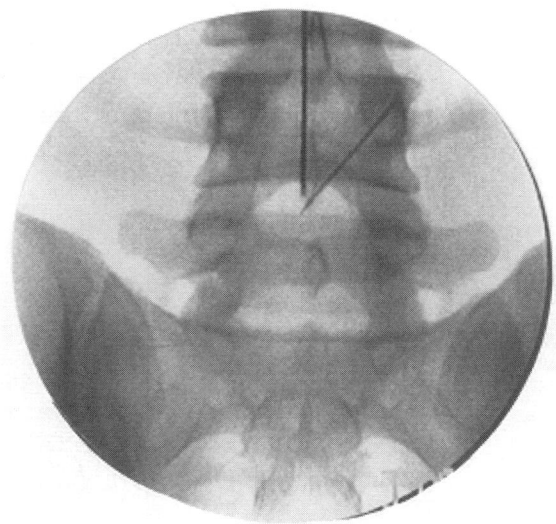

Figure 51.9 *Correct position of the spine.* **Note:** *The spinous process is centered on the spinal body.*

52. FLETCHER SUIT IMPLANT

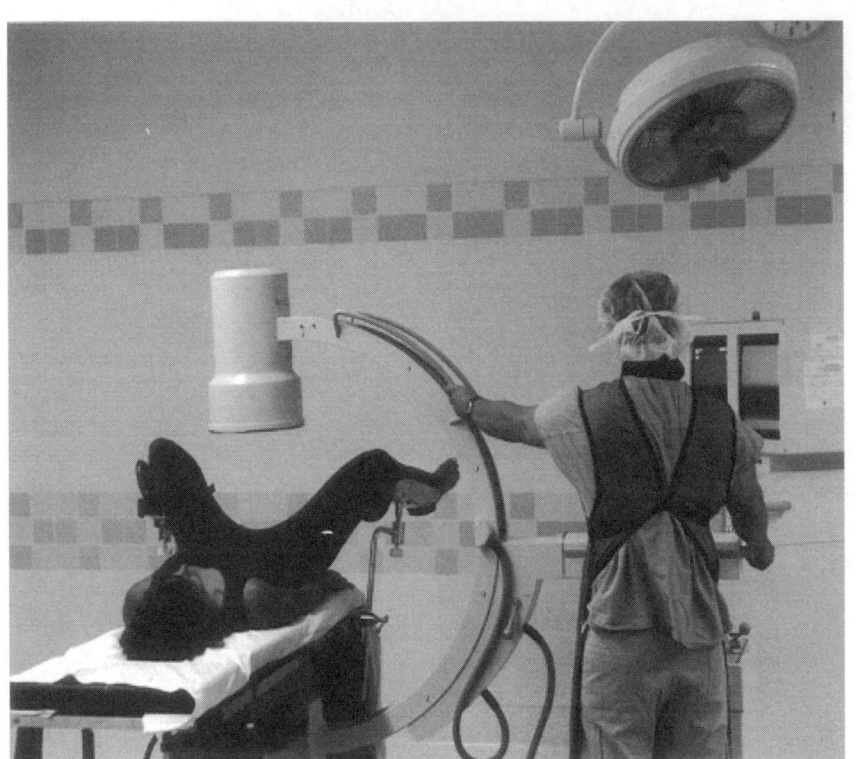

Figure 52.1 *C-arm in ap projection of bladder.*

PATIENT POSITION: Patient will be supine with legs straight or knees slightly bent.

C-ARM POSITION: C-arm will enter perpendicular to patient and in the ap projection.

Notes: Ensure clearance underneath allows for movement from abdomen to the bladder area.

C-arm may have to be slightly rotated over or backward to enhance image of seeds.

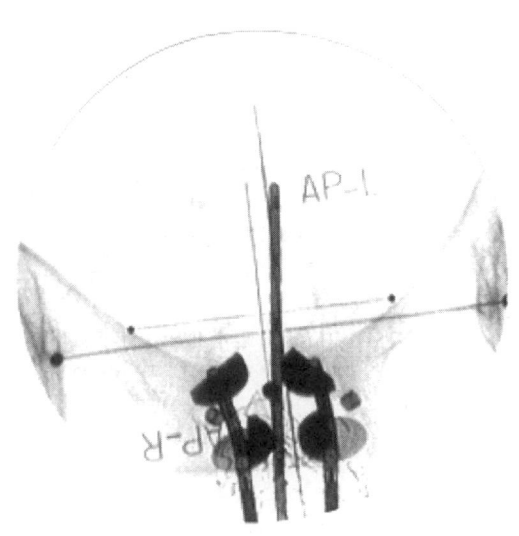

Figure 52.2 *C-arm image of bladder with instrumentation.*

53. RADIOACTIVE SEED IMPLANT

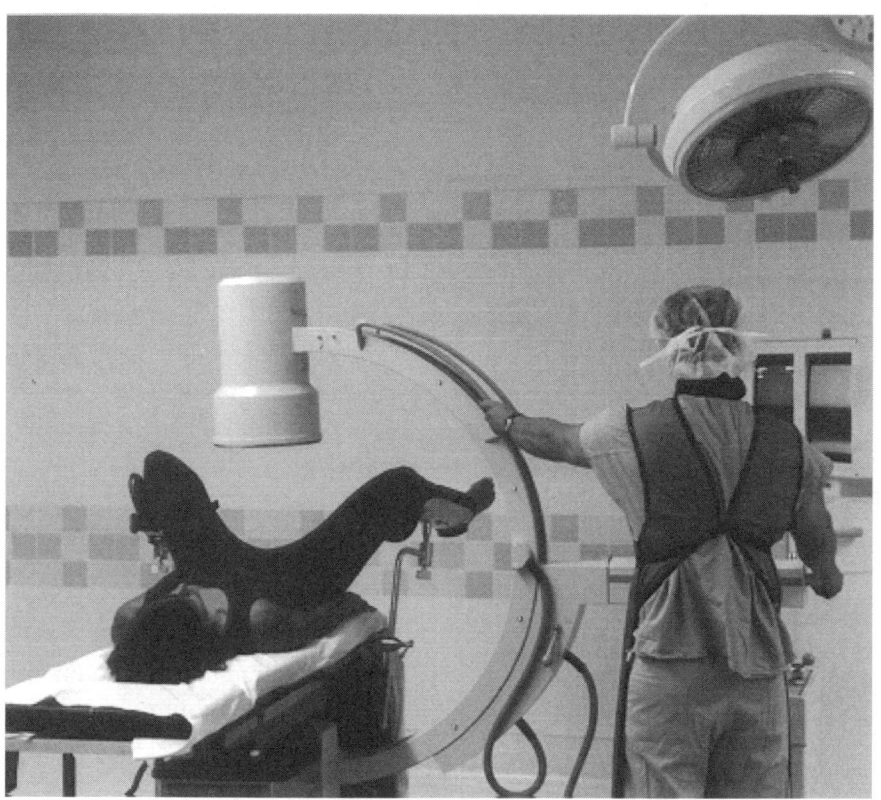

PATIENT POSITION: Patient will be supine with knees flexed toward the chest.

C-ARM POSITION: C-arm will enter in ap projection of abdomen and groin area.

Notes: C-arm should have underneath clearance to allow movement from the abdomen to the groin area.

Decrease object-to-film distance to create a larger field of view.

Figure 53.1 *C-arm in ap projection of abdomen.*

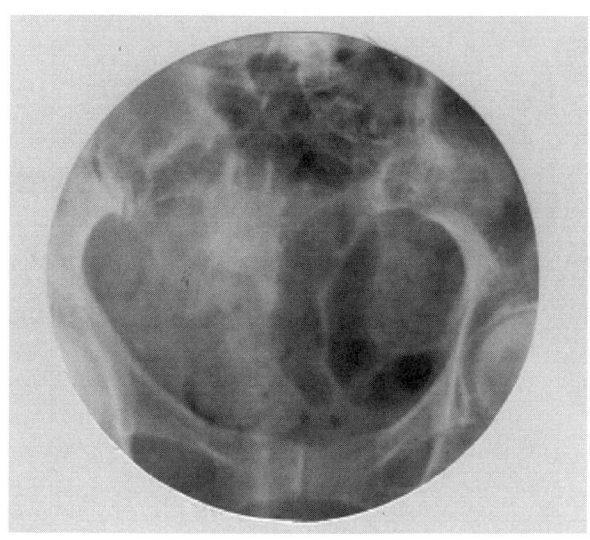

Figure 53.2 *X-ray image of bladder area.*

54. FEMORAL ARTERIOGRAM

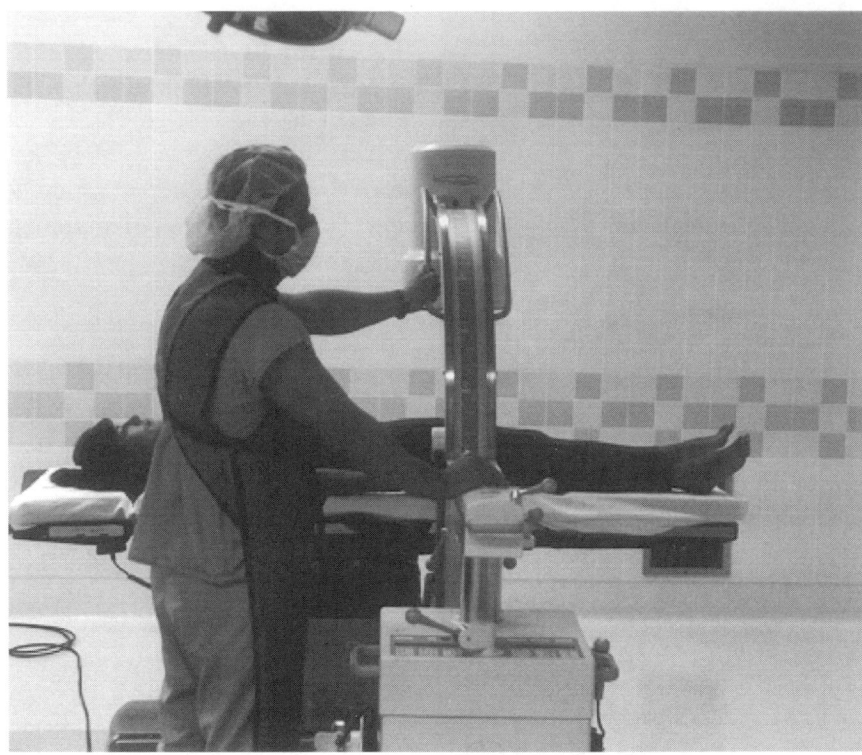

Figure 54.1 *C-arm in ap projection of femur.*

PATIENT POSITION: Patient will be supine with leg externally rotated to throw femoral artery away from femur.

C-ARM POSITION: C-arm will enter in the ap projection of femur.

Notes: Ensure table has room underneath to allow c-arm movement from groin area to the ankle.

C-arm may have to be rotated over or backward to throw artery away from bone.

A subtracted image, or road map image, may be required to enhance the artery.

Table must be radiolucent from groin to the ankle area.

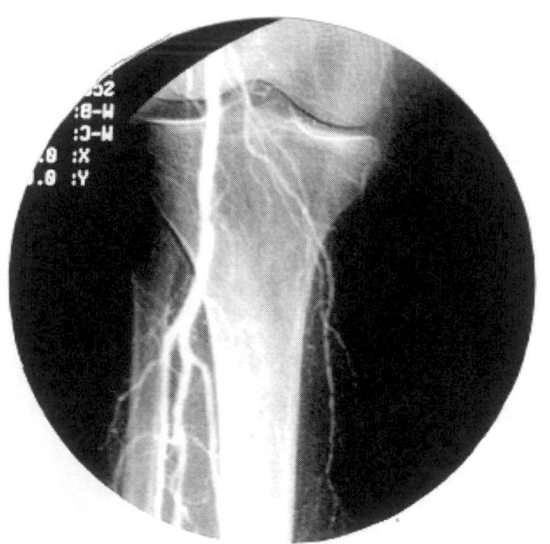

Figure 54.2 *X-ray image of distal femur with contrast media.*

55. PUL

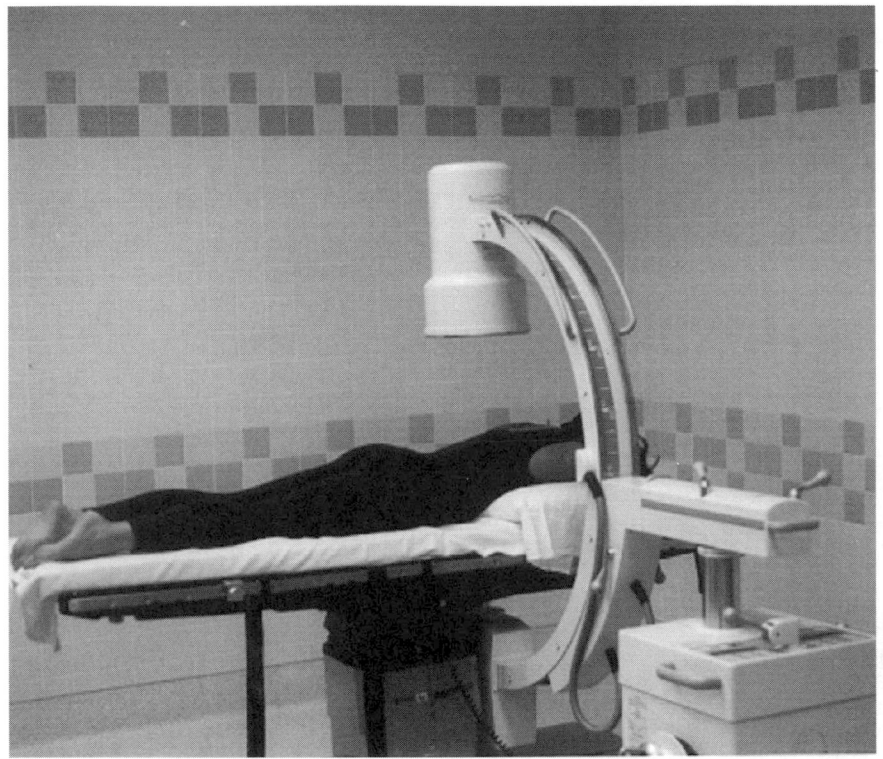

Figure 55.1 *C-arm in pa projection of kidney.*

PATIENT POSITION: Patient will be prone in the right anterior oblique (RAO) or left anterior oblique (LAO) with affected kidney up.

C-ARM POSITION: C-arm will enter perpendicular to patient in the pa projection.

Notes: C-arm may have to be rotated backward to remove spine from view of kidney.

Contrast may be inserted to enhance kidney.

An abdomen or urology mode on C-arm better illustrates this region.

C-arm should have underneath table access from kidney to the bladder.

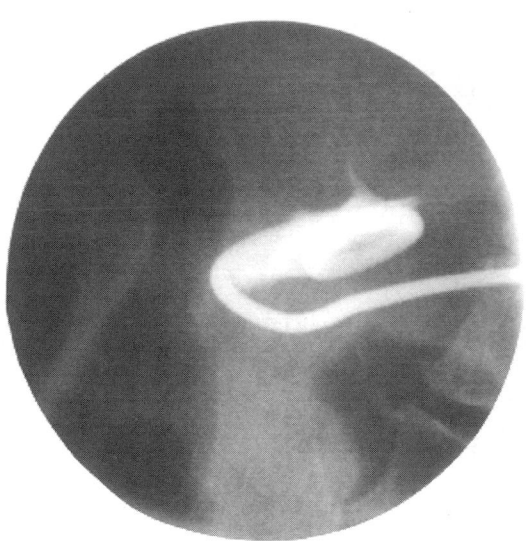

Figure 55.2 *C-arm image of kidney with contrast.*

56. PACEMAKER/A.I.C.D. INSERTION

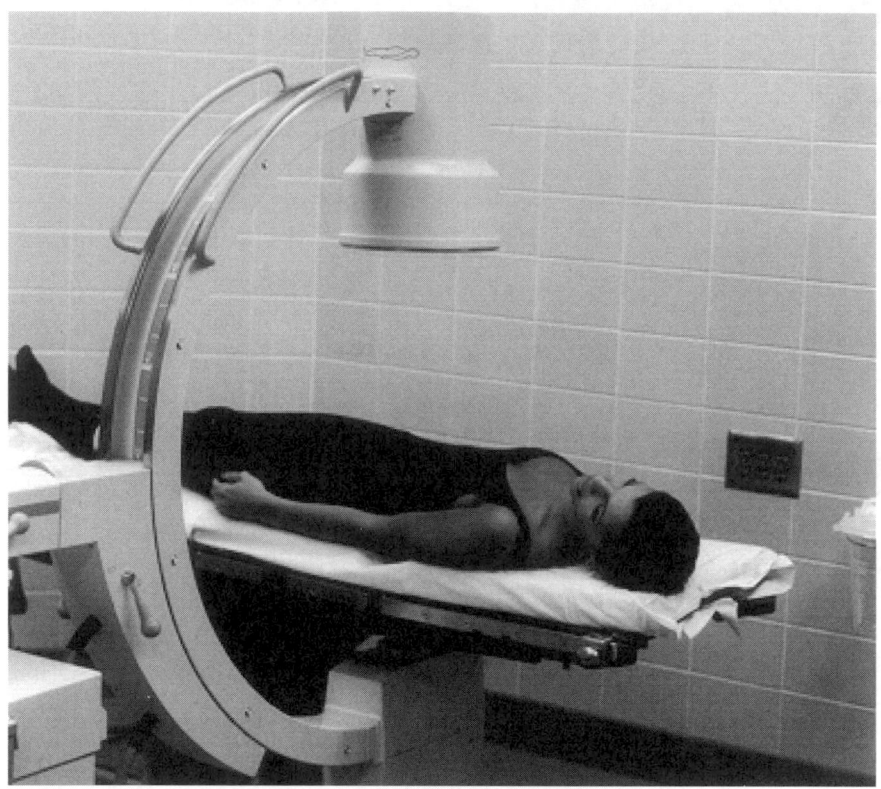

Figure 56.1 *C-arm in ap projection of chest area.*

PATIENT POSITION: Patient will be supine and in slight Trendelenberg.

C-ARM POSITION: C-arm will enter on opposite side of physician in the ap projection.

Notes: Ensure that c-arm has sufficient mobility to follow leads from wound site to apex of heart.

Depending on patient position, the c-arm may have to be rotated 10 to 25 degrees to create RAO view.

A chest program on the c-arm is best utilized for this exam.

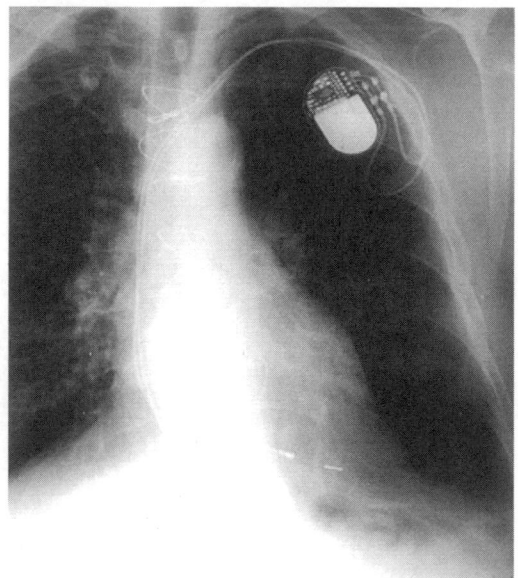

Figure 56.2 *C-arm image of chest area with leads in place.*

57. LAPARASCOPIC CHOLANGIOGRAM

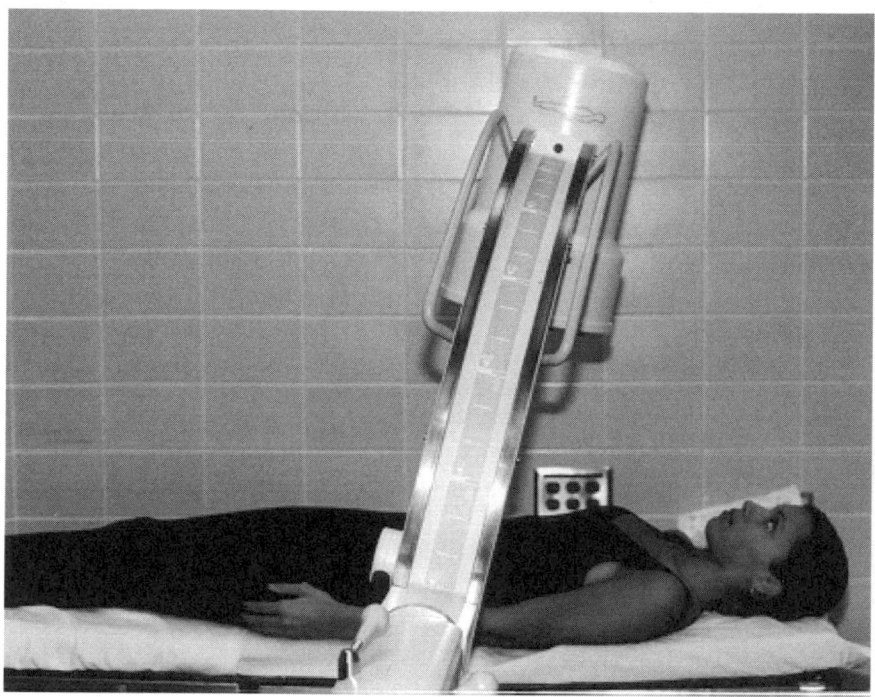

Figure 57.1 *C-arm in ap projection of abdomen.*

PATIENT POSITION: Patient will be supine and tilted slightly toward the left side.

C-ARM POSITION: C-arm will enter the patient in the ap projection and centered over right lower quadrant of the abdomen.

Notes: Patient may have to be tilted in Trendelenberg to ensure filling of ducts.

C-arm may have to be rotated over or backward to place spine out of view of ducts.

Ensure that area underneath table is clear.

Be careful not to dislodge instrumentation protruding from abdomen.

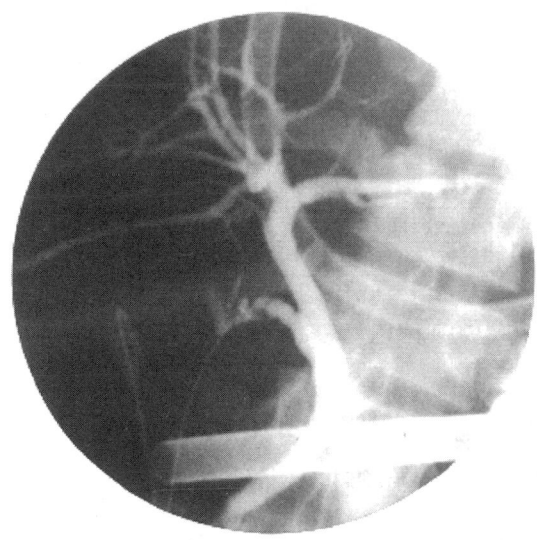

Figure 57.2 *C-arm image of cholangiogram.*

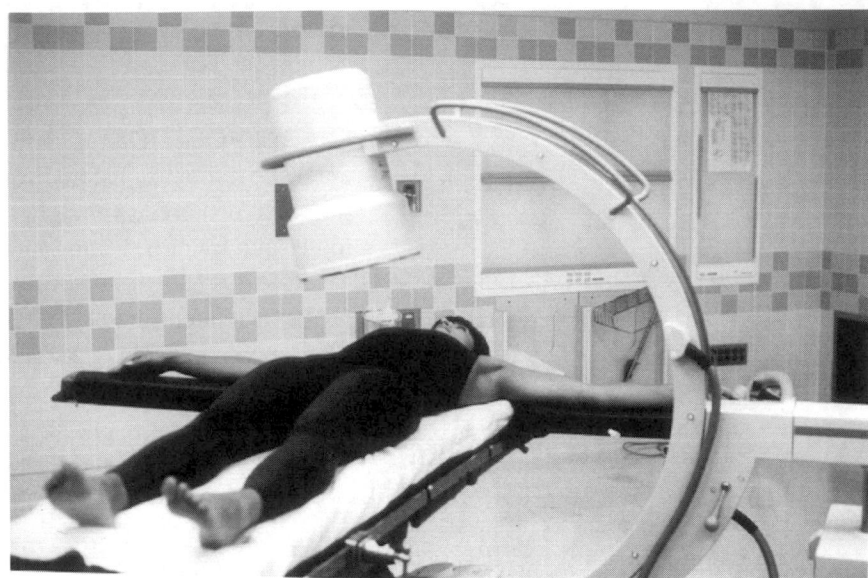

Figure 57.3 *The c-arm is rotated over the top during a laparascopic cholangiogram. This will throw the duct away from the spine for better visualization.*

58. GREENFELD FILTER PLACEMENT

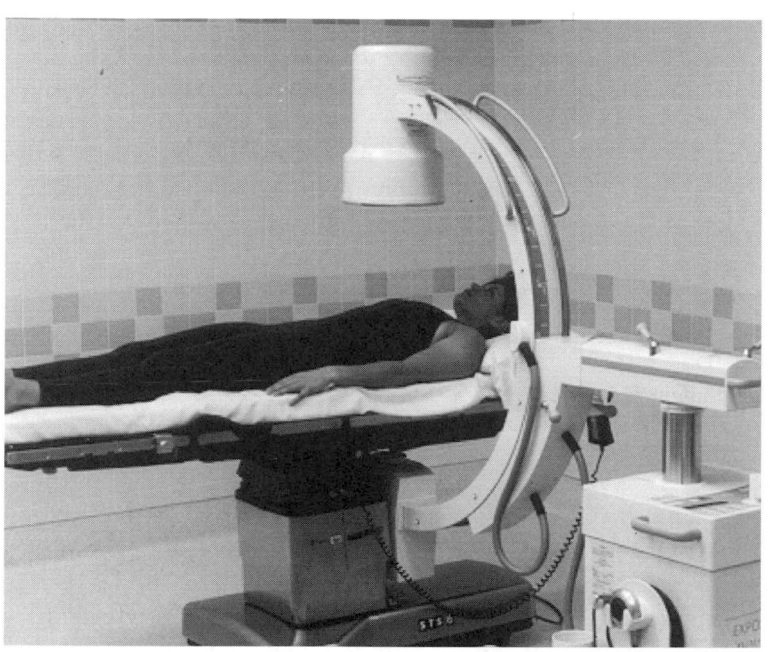

PATIENT POSITION: Patient will be supine and on a radiolucent table.

C-ARM POSITION: C-arm will enter perpendicular to the patient and in the ap projection.

Notes: Ensure patient is positioned to allow the c-arm to scan from chest area to the groin.

Area underneath table should be clear to allow movement of c-arm.

C-arm may have to be rotated over or backward to throw filter out of alignment with spine.

Figure 58.1 *C-arm in ap projection of abdomen.*

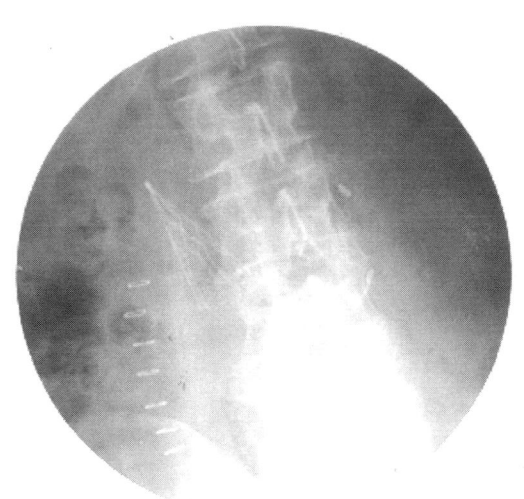

Figure 58.2 *X-ray image of abdomen with filter in place.*

59. STAPLE HEMI-EPIPHYSIODESIS
(AP POSITION)

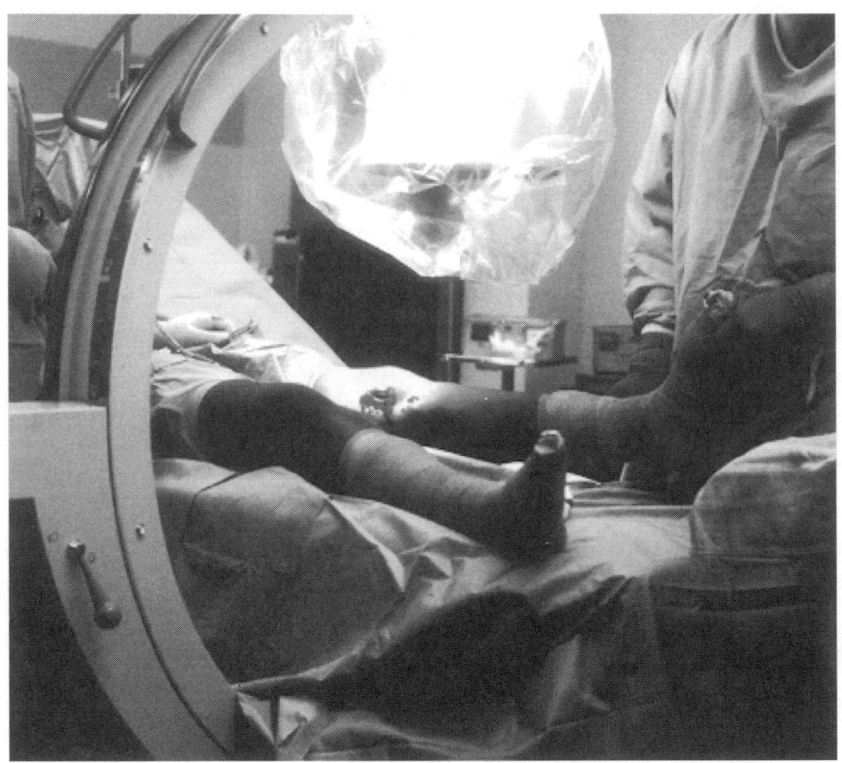

PATIENT POSITION: Patient will be supine with the lower extremities on a radiolucent table.

C-ARM POSITION: C-arm will enter perpendicular to the patient and on the opposite side of the surgeon.

Notes: Metallic marker may be used to locate growth plate position.

C-arm may have to be rotated and tilted in line with the flexed and externally rotated leg to obtain a true lateral of the knee.

C-arm should be covered with sterile drape when working over a sterile field.

Figure 59.1 *C-arm in ap projection of affected knee.*

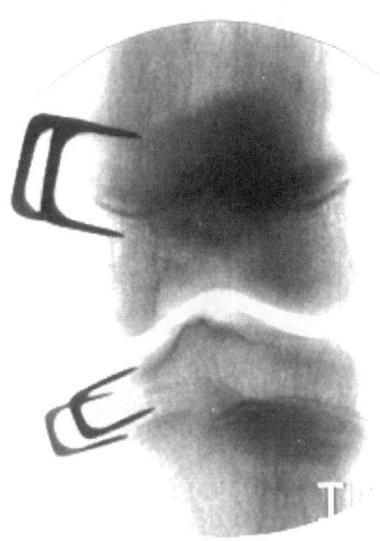

Figure 59.2 *X-ray image of affected knee ap view.*

60. STAPLE HEMI-EPIPHYSIODESIS
(LATERAL POSITION)

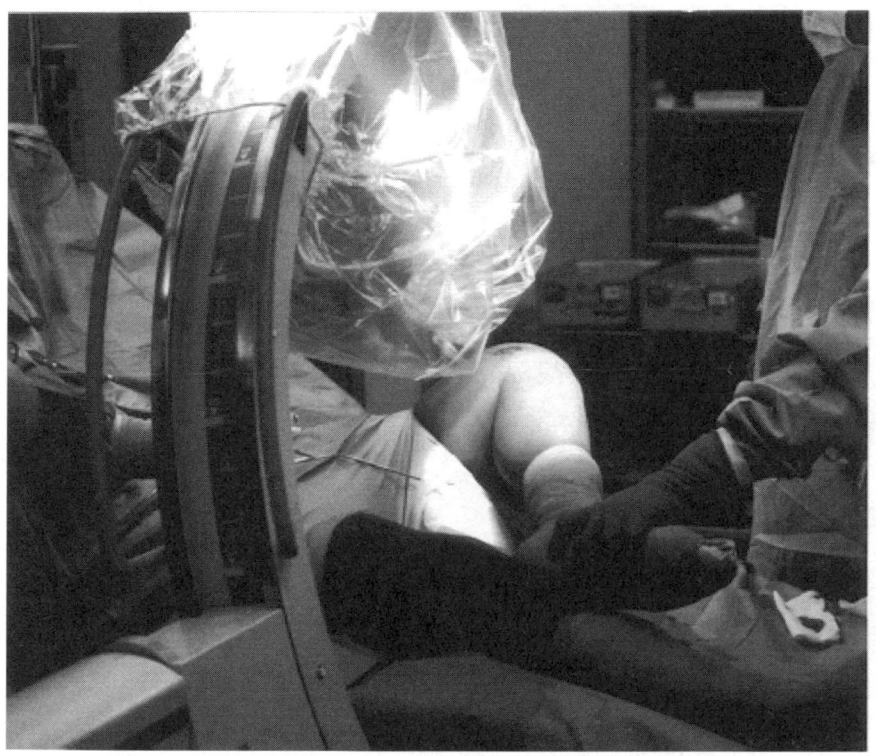

Figure 60.1 *C-arm in lateral projection of affected knee.*

PATIENT POSITION:
Patient will be supine with the lower extremities on a radiolucent table. The leg will be flexed and externally rotated to view the lateral profile of the knee.

C-ARM POSITION: C-arm will enter perpendicular to the patient and on the opposite side of the surgeon. C-arm will have to be tilted and rotated to align with the lateral profile of the knee.

Notes: Procedure may be done on the medial or lateral aspect of the knee. It may also be performed medial and lateral simultaneously.

The knee should be positioned beyond or within the lateral edge of the table to avoid the radiopaque rim of table.

C-arm should be covered with sterile drape when working over a sterile field.

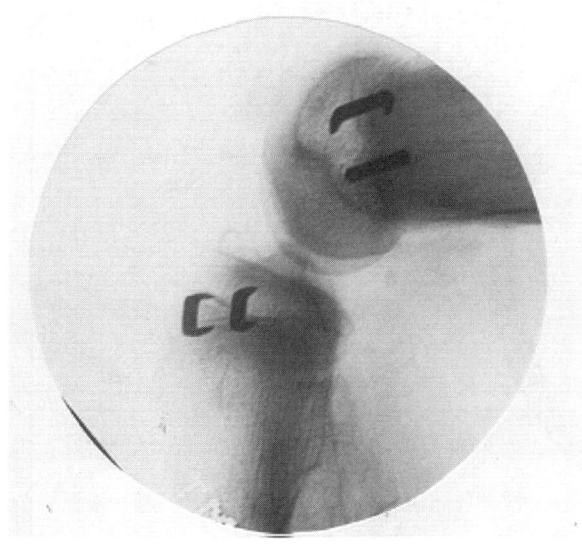

Figure 60.2 *X-ray image of affected knee lateral view.*

61. HIP ARTHROGRAM
(AP VIEW)

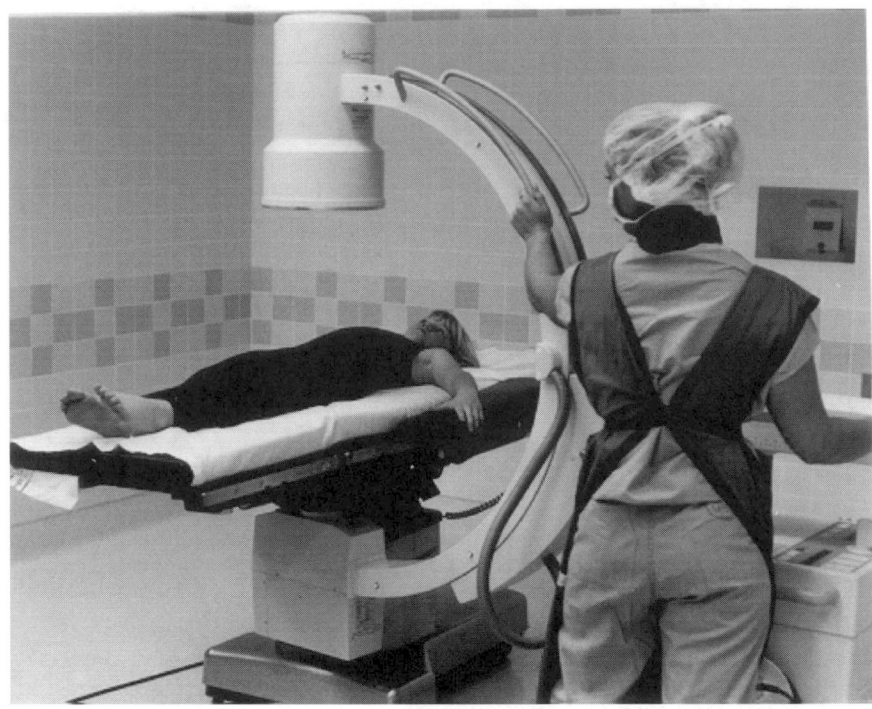

PATIENT POSITION: Patient will be supine with the legs extended. Legs may be crossed to expose affected hip.

C-ARM POSITION: C-arm will enter perpendicular to the patient and in the ap projection.

Notes: Ensure that patient's hips are on radiolucent portion of the table.

C-arm may have to be rotated over or backward to view different aspects of the hip

Hip may have to be abducted to view contrast with the c-arm in different position.

Figure 61.1 C-arm in ap projection of the affected hip.

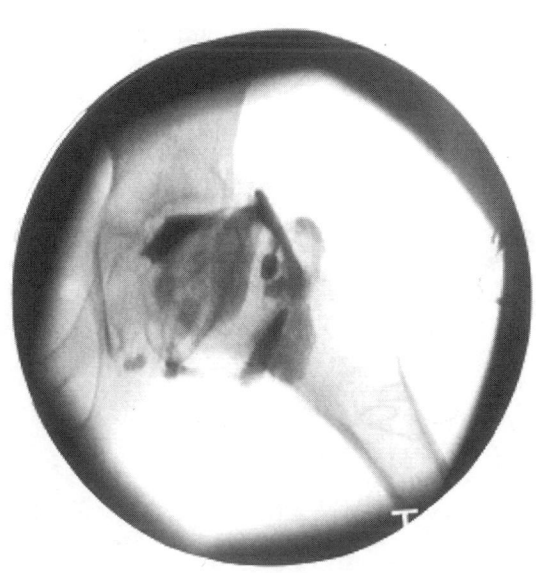

Figure 61.2 X-ray image of the affected hip.

62. HIP ARTHROGRAM
(LATERAL VIEW)

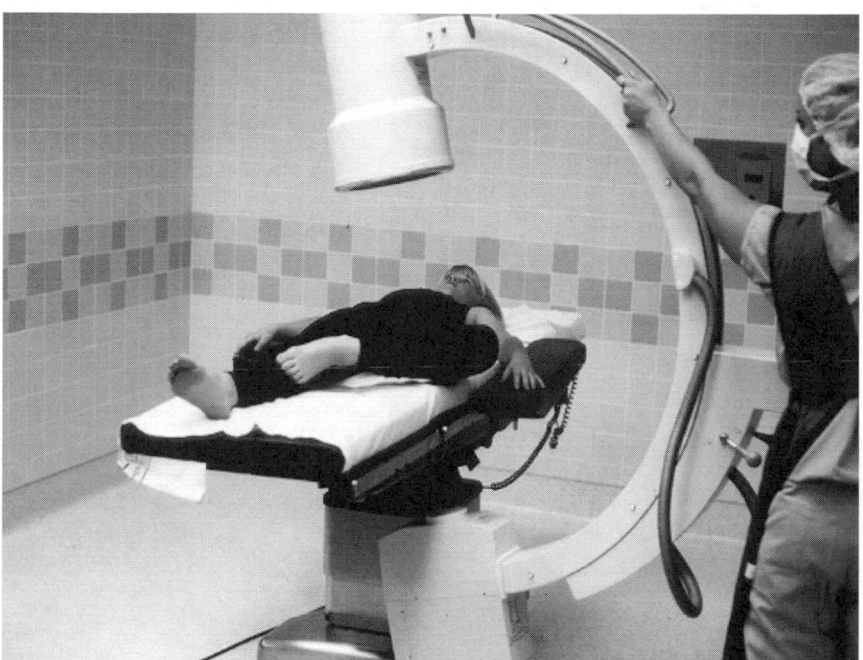

PATIENT POSITION: Patient will be supine with the affected hip in the frog-leg position.

C-ARM POSITION: C-arm will enter in the ap projection and may have to be rotated over or backward to view different aspects of the hip.

Notes: Physician will assist in positioning the patient in the frog-leg position.

The hip may be crossed or abducted to view the hip in a stressed position.

Figure 62.1 *C-arm in ap projection of the hip, which is in the frog-leg position.*

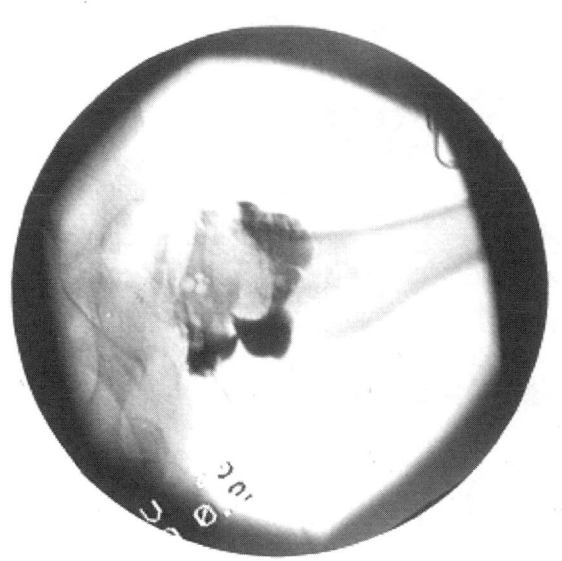

Figure 62.2 *X-ray image of lateral view of the hip.*

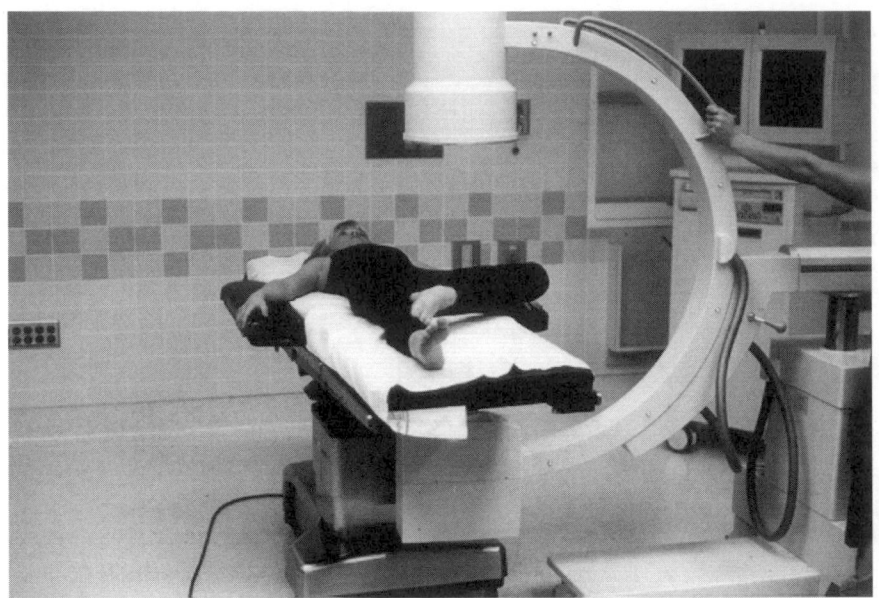

Figure 62.3 *The affected leg may be frogged to better view the hip joint. This illustration shows the hip in that position.*

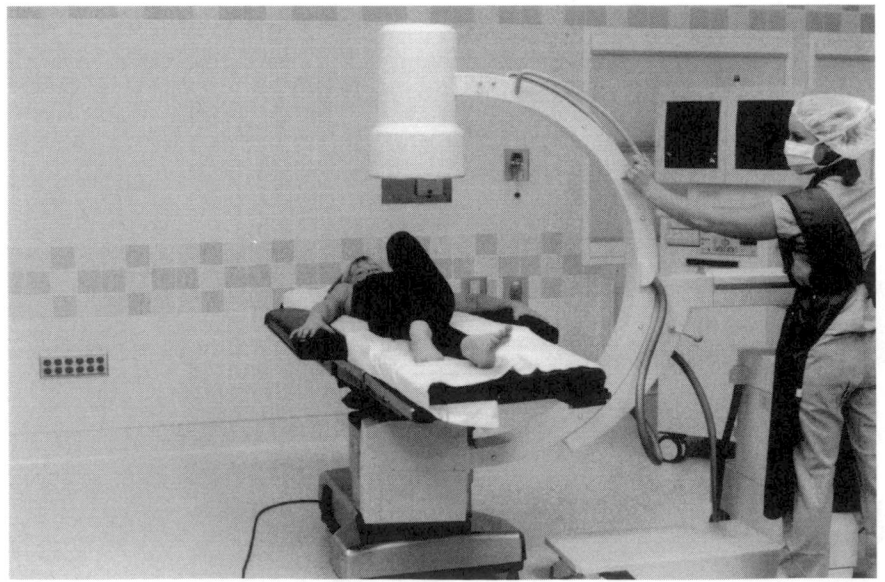

Figure 62.4 *To better view the out spacing of the hip the affected leg can be positioned across the unaffected leg, as shown in this illustration.*

Part II:
Intra-Operative Examinations

63. INTRA-OPERATIVE SKULL
(AP VIEW)

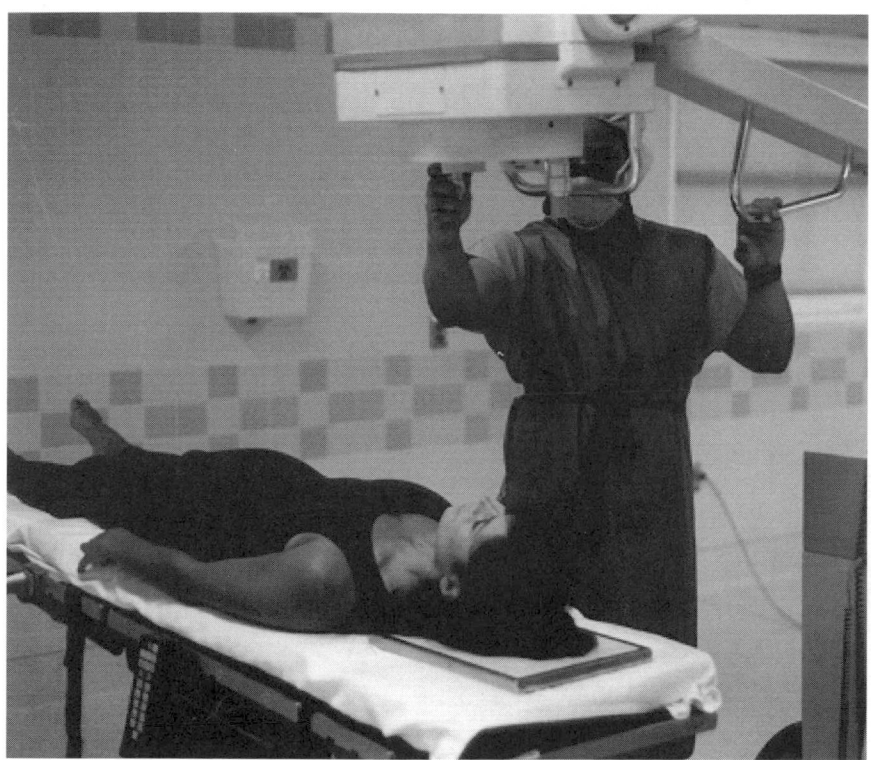

PATIENT POSITION: Patient will be in the supine or with head and shoulder slightly elevated.

X-RAY MACHINE: Portable x-ray will enter in the ap projection of the skull.

Notes: Grid cassette must have sterile cover when working on sterile field.

Position X-ray beam perpendicular to grid cassette and patient's skull.

Patient's skull or the x-ray beam may have to be manipulated to project a true ap view.

Figure 63.1 *X-ray machine and patient positioned for ap view of skull.*

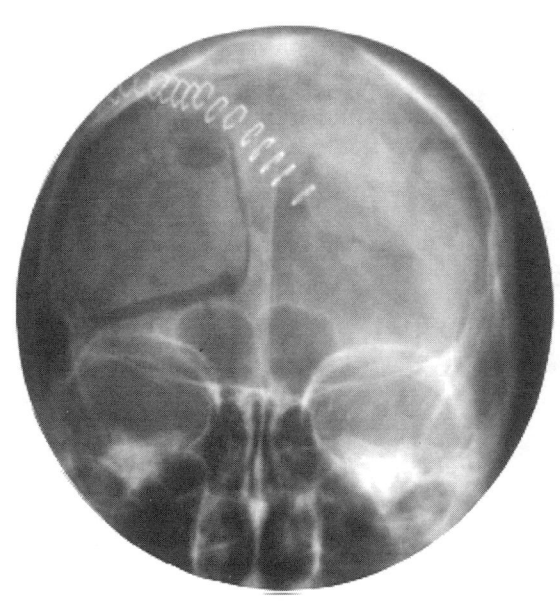

Figure 63.2 *X-ray image of ap skull.*

64. INTRA-OPERATIVE SKULL
(LATERAL VIEW)

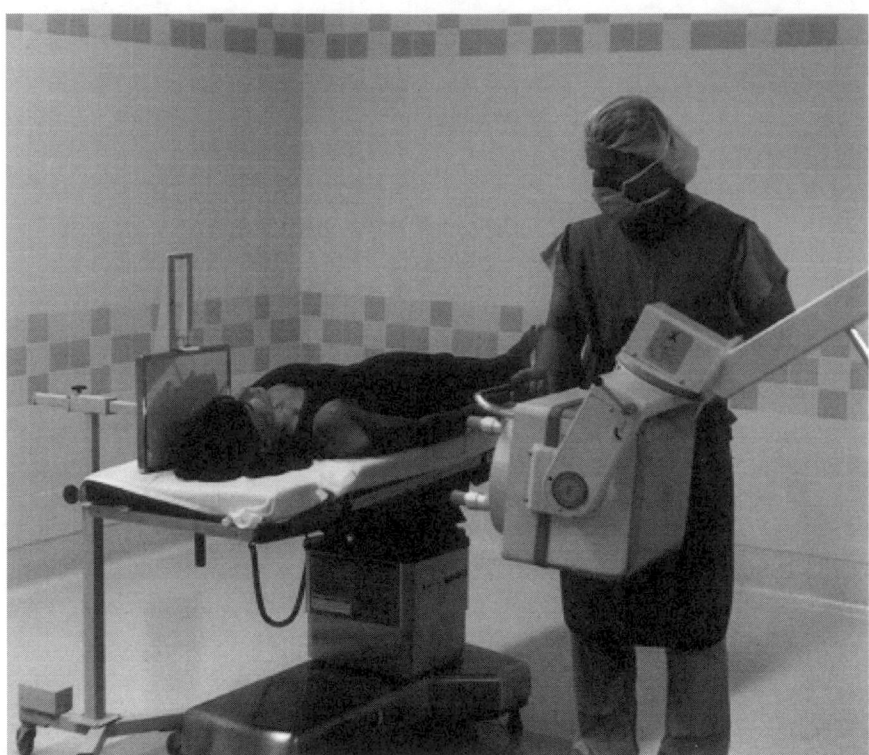

Figure 64.1 *X-ray machine and grid cassette positioned for lateral view of skull.*

PATIENT POSITION: Patient will be supine or with head and shoulders slightly elevated.

X-RAY MACHINE: Portable X-ray will enter lateral and perpendicular to the patient.

Notes: Place grid cassette along side and parallel to patient's skull.

Position X-ray beam on line and perpendicular to patient's skull.

Cover grid cassette with sterile drape if working on sterile field.

Ensure X-ray beam is parallel to the floor.

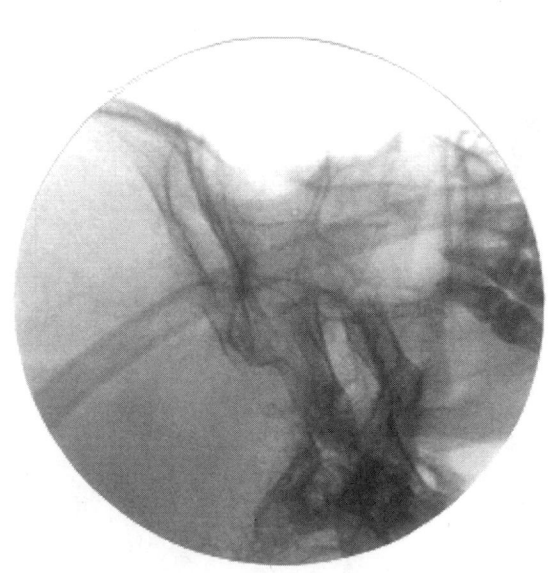

Figure 64.2 *X-ray image of lateral skull.*

65. INTRA-OPERATIVE SHOULDER
(AP VIEW)

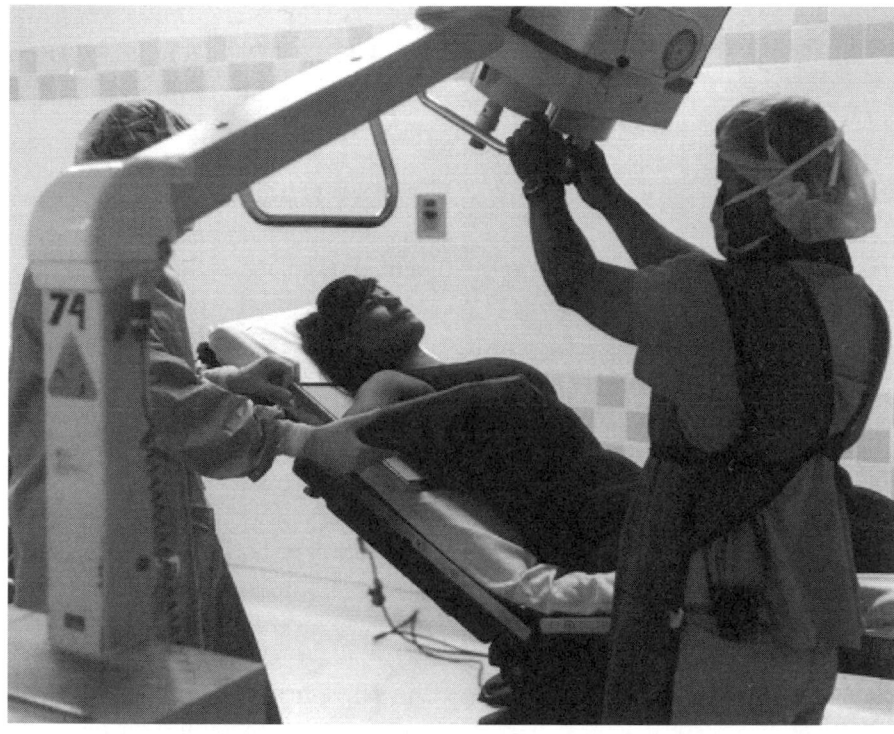

PATIENT POSITION: Patient will be supine or in the sitting position.

X-RAY MACHINE: Portable X-ray will enter lateral to the patient.

Notes: Physician will place cassette posterior to the patient and in line with X-ray beam to obtain a true ap of the shoulder.

Position X-ray beam to obtain a true ap of the shoulder.

X-ray tube will have to be covered with sterile cover before placing over sterile field.

Figure 65.1 *X-ray machine and patient positioned for ap view of shoulder.*

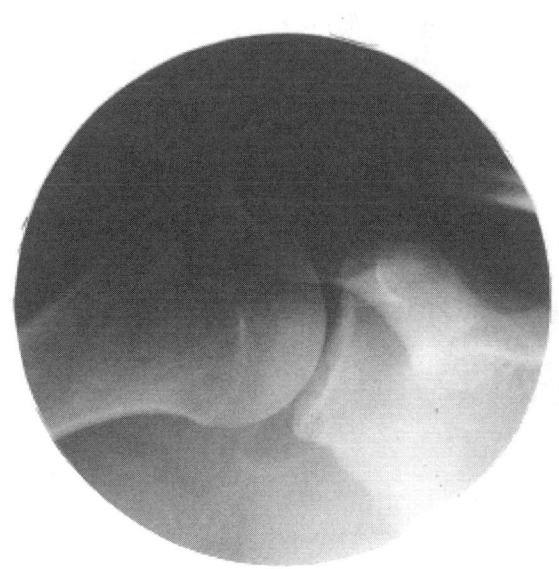

Figure 65.2 *X-ray image of ap shoulder.*

66. INTRA-OPERATIVE SHOULDER
(AXILLARY VIEW)

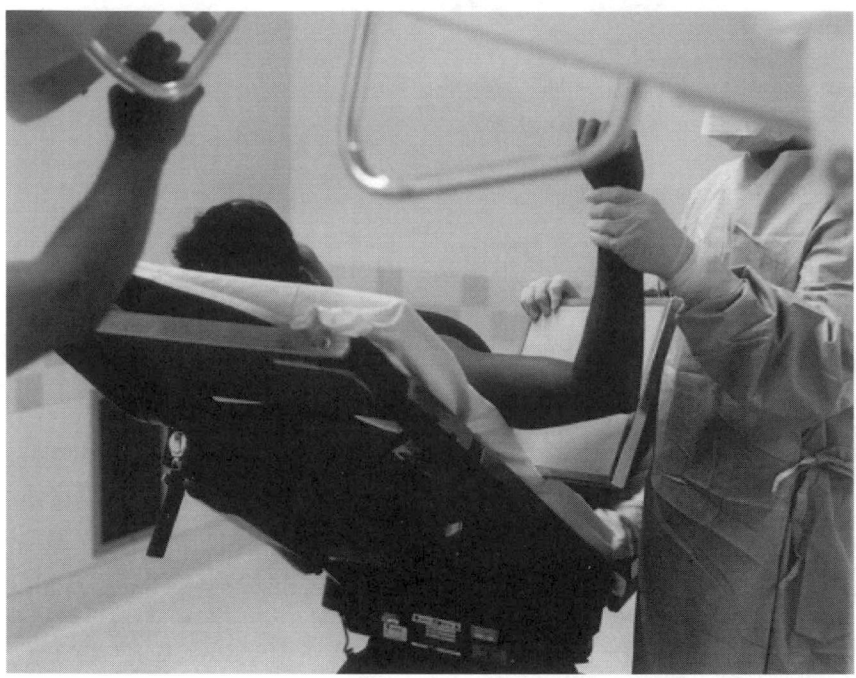

Figure 66.1 *X-ray machine and patient positioned for axillary view of shoulder.*

PATIENT POSITION: Patient will be supine or in the sitting position.

X-RAY MACHINE: Portable X-ray will enter lateral to the patient and on the side of the affected shoulder.

Notes: Cover cassette with sterile cover before placing on sterile field.

Physician will place cassette under shoulder to obtain the axillary view.

Cover X-ray tube with sterile cover before placing over field.

X-ray tube may have to be angled laterally to align with cassette to create the axillary view.

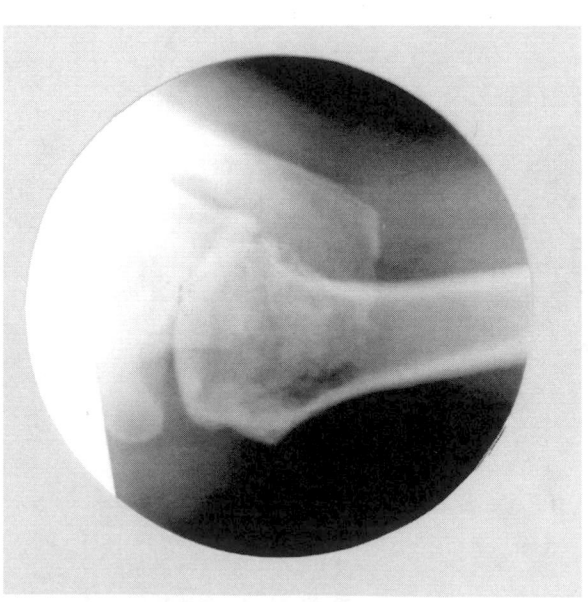

Figure 66.2 *X-ray image of shoulder axillary view.*

67. INTRA-OPERATIVE ELBOW
(PA VIEW)

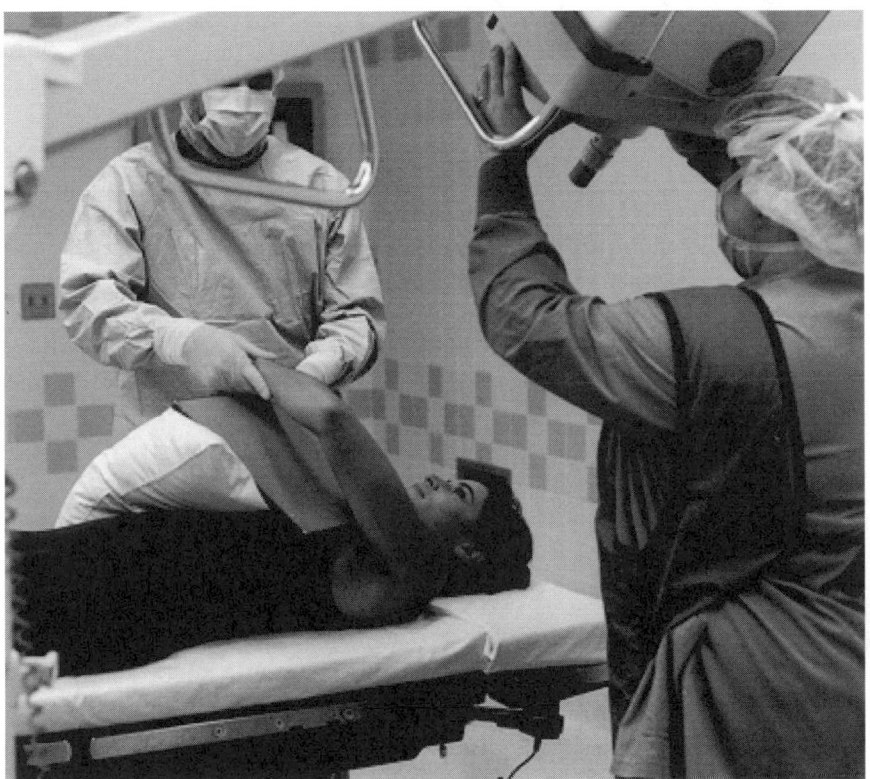

Figure 67.1 *X-ray machine and patient positioned for view of elbow pa.*

PATIENT POSITION: Patient will be supine with the affected elbow positioned across the body or extended upward.

X-RAY MACHINE: Portable X-ray machine will enter lateral to the patient and on the affected elbow side.

Notes: Cover cassette with sterile cover before placing on the field.

Physician will place cassette in proper position on the field.

Cover X-ray tube with sterile cover before placing on the field.

Angle X-ray tube perpendicular to cassette and in line with elbow to create a true lateral view.

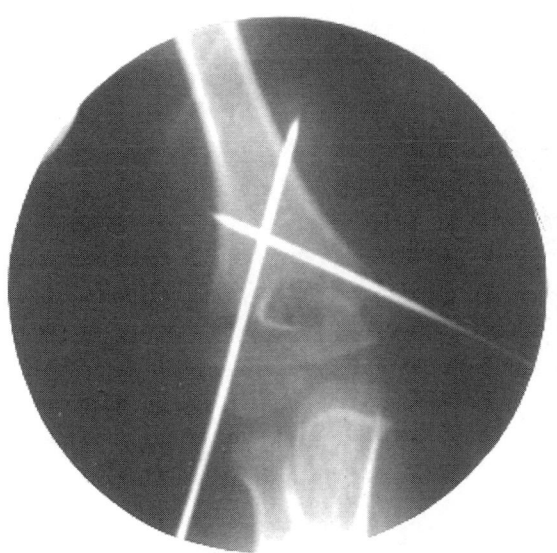

Figure 67.2 *X-ray image of pa elbow with pins inserted.*

68. INTRA-OPERATIVE ELBOW
(LATERAL VIEW)

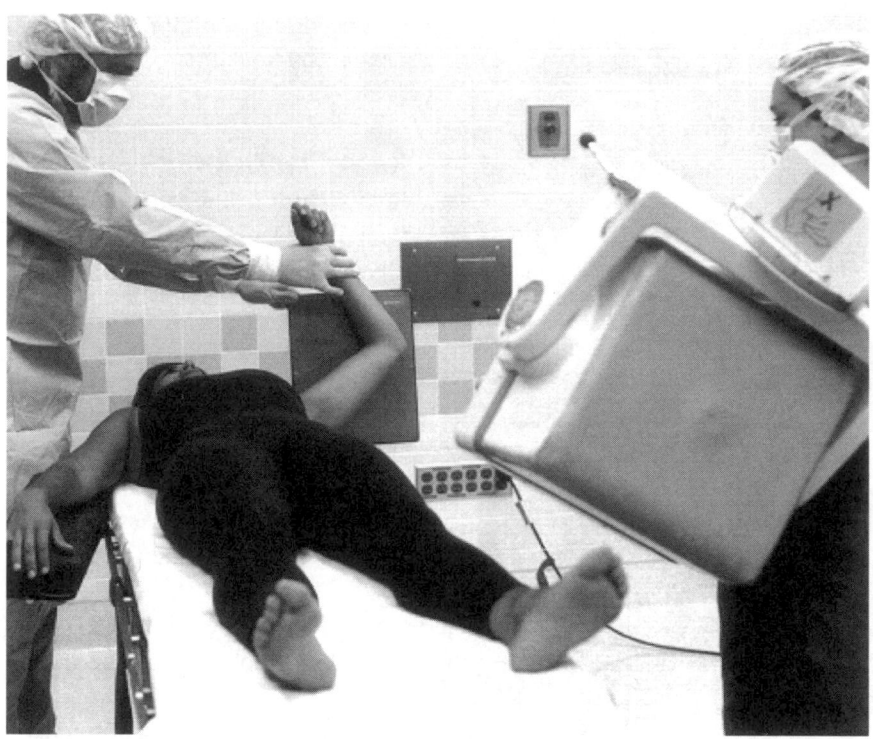

PATIENT POSITION: Patient will be supine with the affected elbow bent toward the body.

X-RAY MACHINE: Portable X-ray machine will enter parallel to the patient's head or at the feet.

Notes: Cover X-ray tube with sterile cover when positioning over field.

Angle the beam to create a true lateral view.

Patient's arms may have to be raised or lowered to assist with obtaining a true lateral view.

Figure 68.1 *X-ray machine and patient's elbow positioned for lateral view of elbow.*

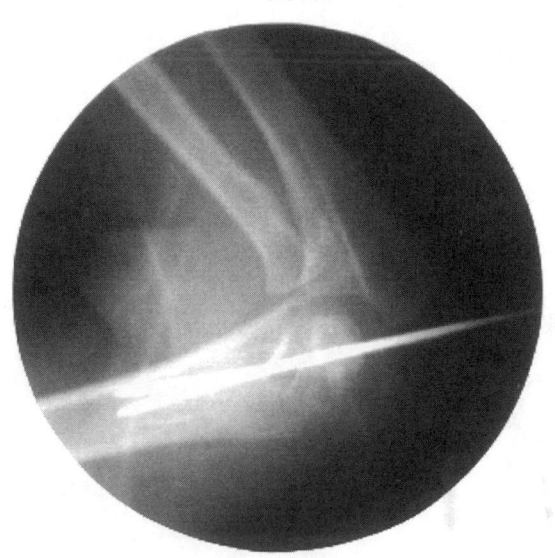

Figure 68.2 *X-ray image of lateral elbow with pins inserted.*

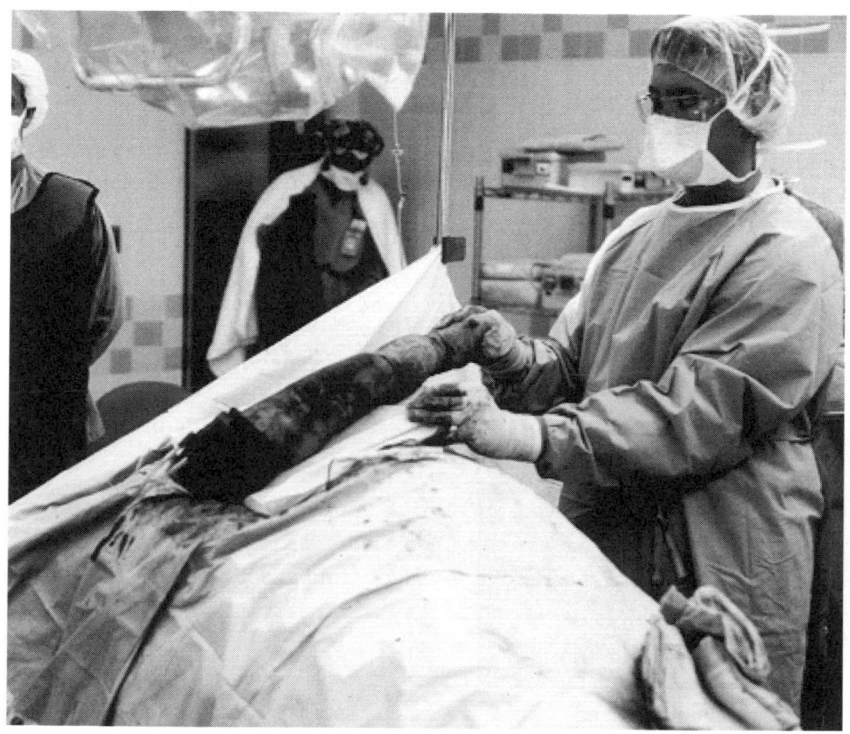

Figure 68.3 *Intra-op pa view of the elbow being performed. When taking this view, turn the palm downward. This will rotate the radial head and promote a true pa view of the elbow.*

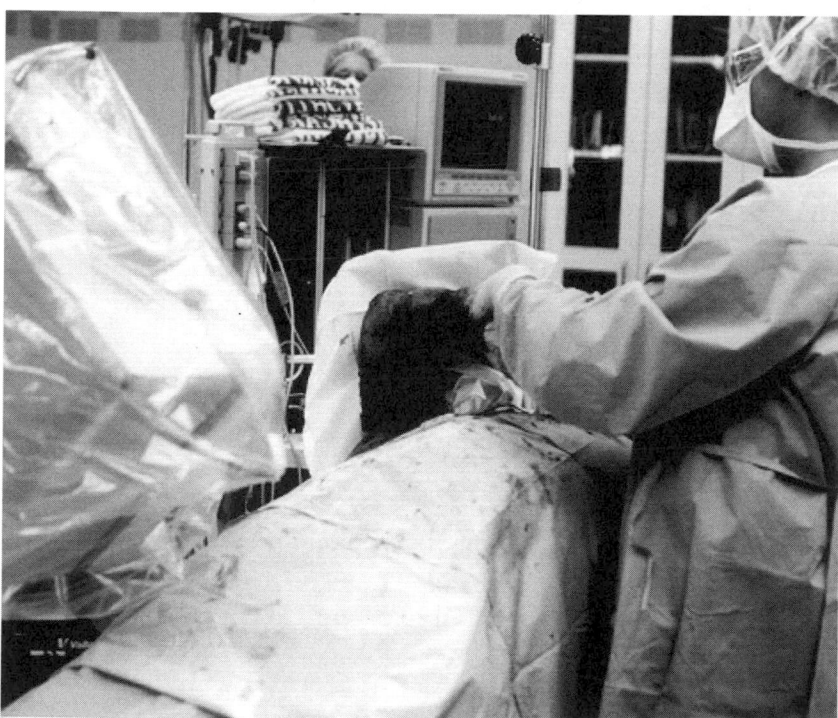

Figure 68.4 *When taking the lateral view of the elbow intra-op, the palm should face downward, rotating the radial head to promote a true lateral of the elbow.*

69. INTRA-OPERATIVE WRIST
(AP USING FINGERTRAPS)

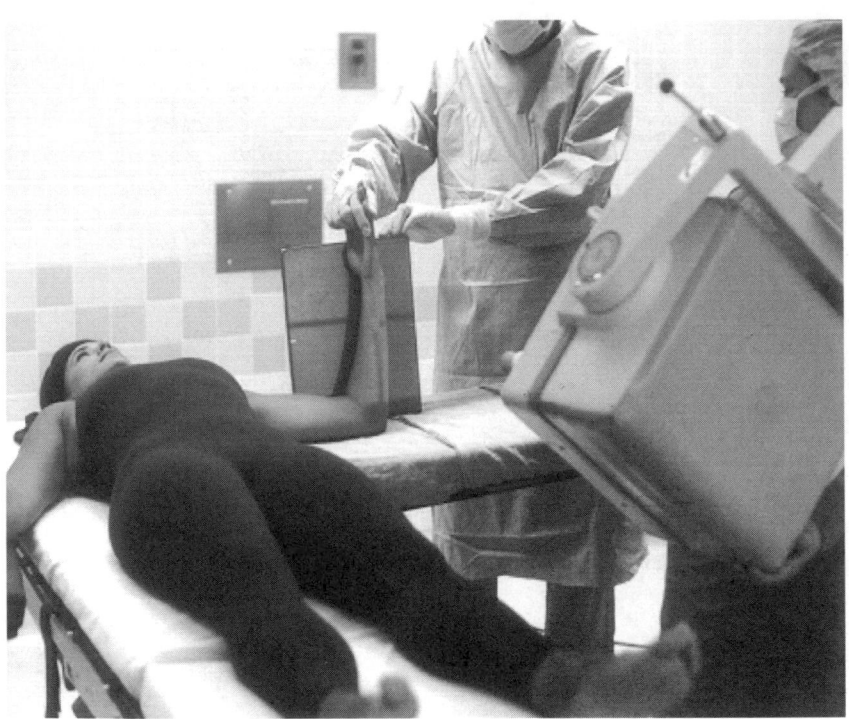

PATIENT POSITION: Patient will be in the supine position with the affected wrist skyward in fingertraps.

X-RAY MACHINE: Portable X-ray will enter in the ap or pa plane with the beam parallel to the floor.

Notes: Upright grid holder may have to be used.

Cover cassette with sterile cover if working on sterile field.

For lateral view position portable X-ray and cassette to obtain view.

Figure 69.1 *X-ray machine and patient positioned for ap wrist.*

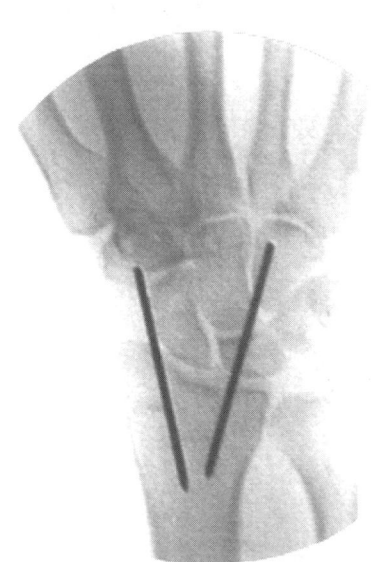

Figure 69.2 *X-ray image of ap wrist with pins inserted.*

70. INTRA-OPERATIVE WRIST
(LATERAL USING FINGERTRAPS)

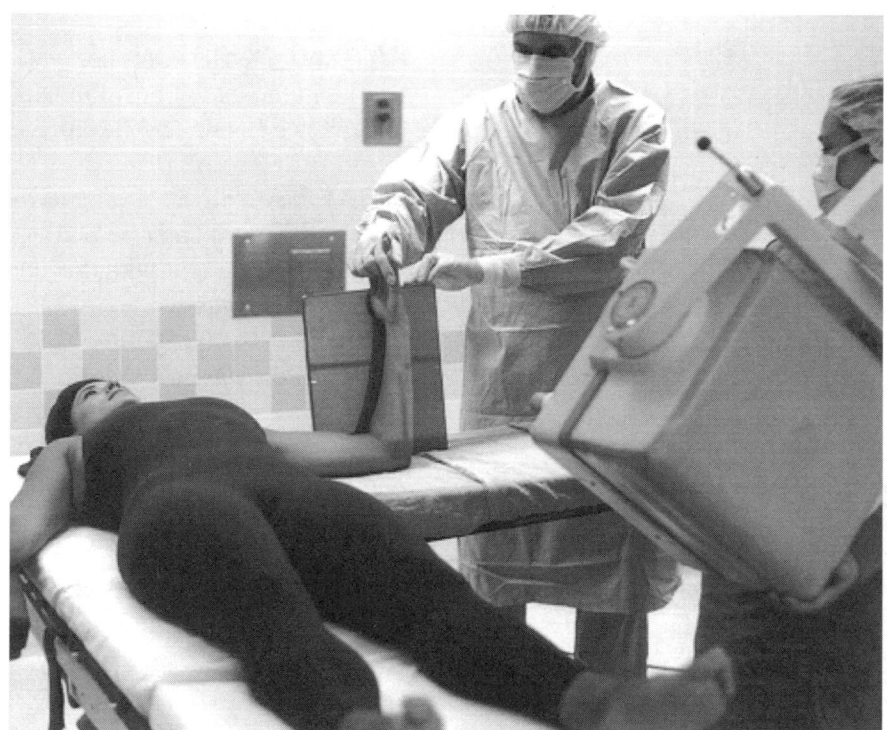

PATIENT POSITION: Patient will be in the supine position with the affected wrist skyward in fingertraps.

X-RAY MACHINE: Portable x-ray will enter perpendicular to the wrist with the beam parallel to the floor.

Notes: Upright grid holder may have to be used.

Cover cassette with sterile cover if working on sterile field.

Wrist may have to be manipulated to create a true lateral view.

Figure 70.1 *X-ray machine and patient positioned for lateral view of wrist.*

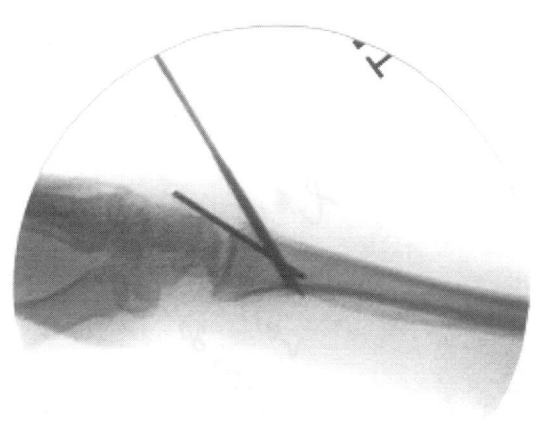

Figure 70.2 *X-ray image of lateral wrist with pins.*

71. INTRA-OPERATIVE FROG-LEG HIP
(CROSS TABLE AP VIEW)

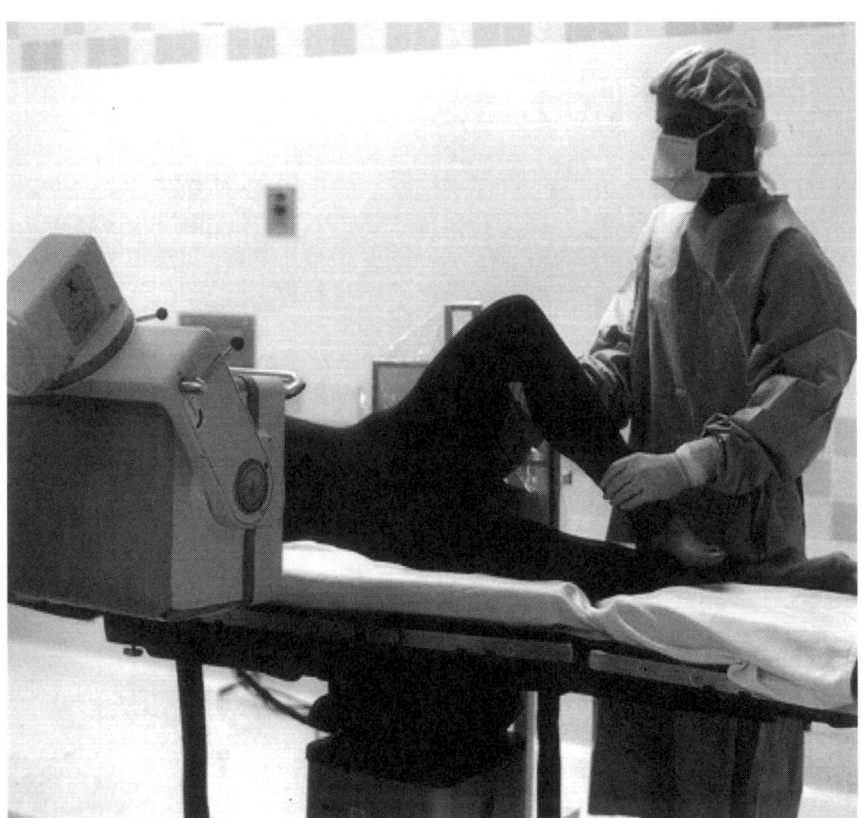

Figure 71.1 *X-ray machine and patient positioned for lateral frog leg hip view.*

PATIENT POSITION: Patient will be in the lateral position with the affected leg up and flexed.

X-RAY MACHINE: Portable X-ray machine will enter perpendicular to the patient with the tube parallel to floor.

Notes: Position grid cassette along side and parallel to patient.

X-ray beam should be on line and perpendicular to the hip.

Cover grid cassette with sterile drape if working on sterile field.

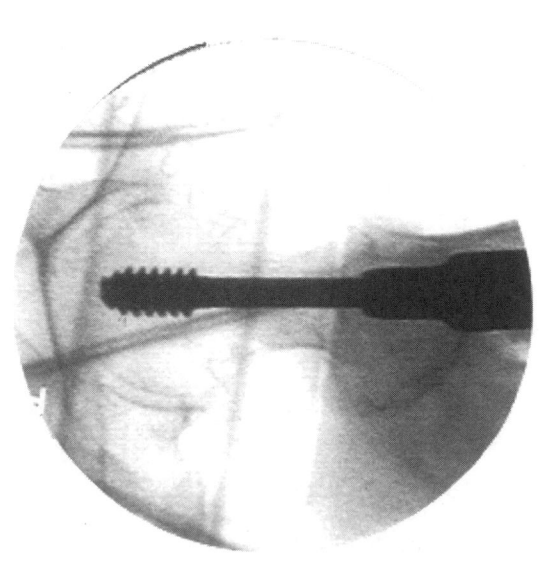

Figure 71.2 *X-ray image of lateral hip.*

72. INTRA-OPERATIVE PELVIS AP
(PATIENT IN LATERAL POSITION)

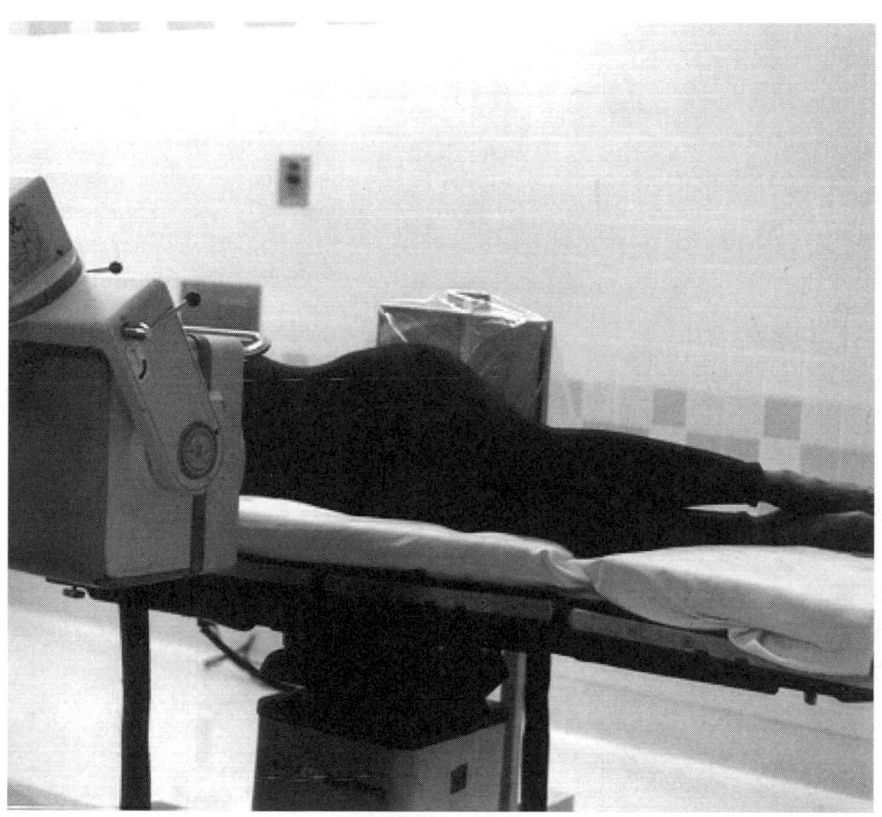

Figure 72.1 *X-ray machine and cassette positioned for cross-table lateral pelvis.*

PATIENT POSITION: Patient will be in the lateral position with affected hip up.

X-RAY MACHINE: Portable x-ray will enter with the beam perpendicular to patient.

Notes: Place grid cassette on opposite side of x-ray machine and in line with the beam.

If working on sterile field grid cassette will have to be covered with sterile drape.

Ensure grid cassette is perpendicular to beam. Beam should be parallel to the floor.

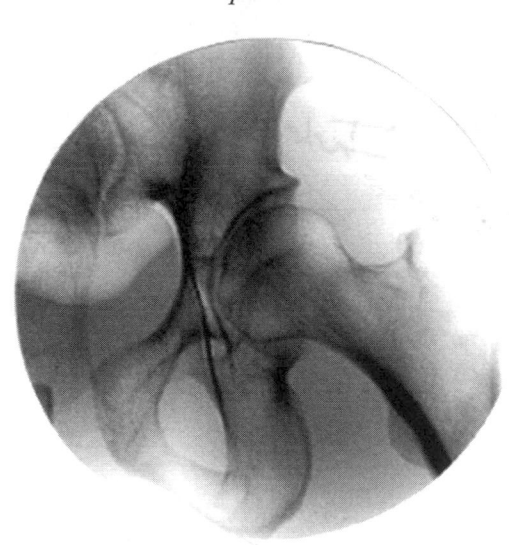

Figure 72..2 *X-ray image of ap pelvis.*

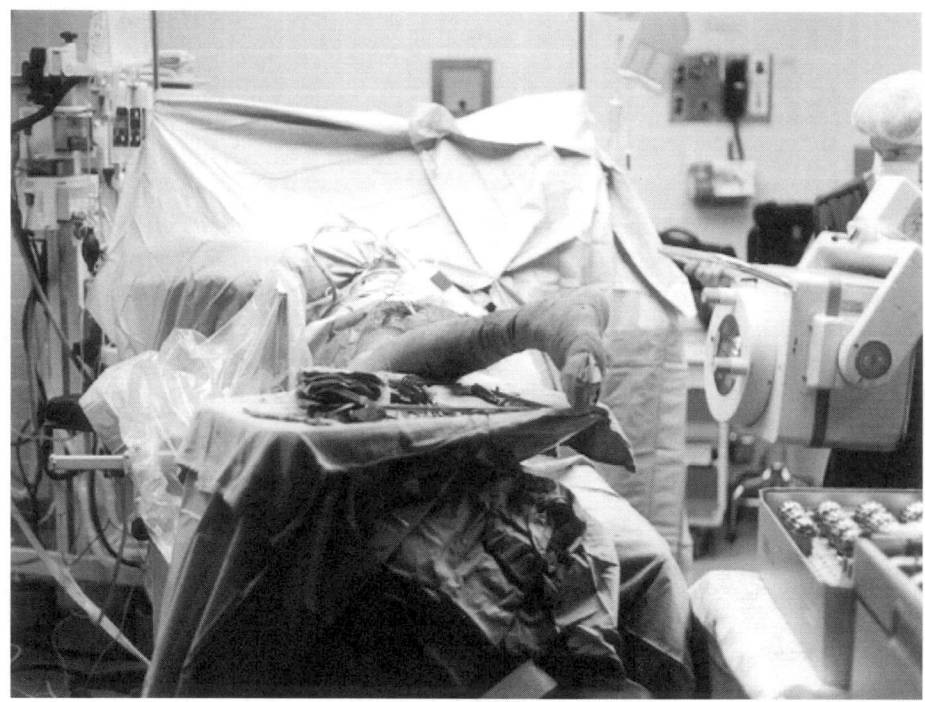

Figure 72.3 Incorrect positioning of the femur when shooting a cross-table view of the hip. Note that the knee is pointed downward. This causes the femur to rotate and will not give a true ap or pa view of the hip.

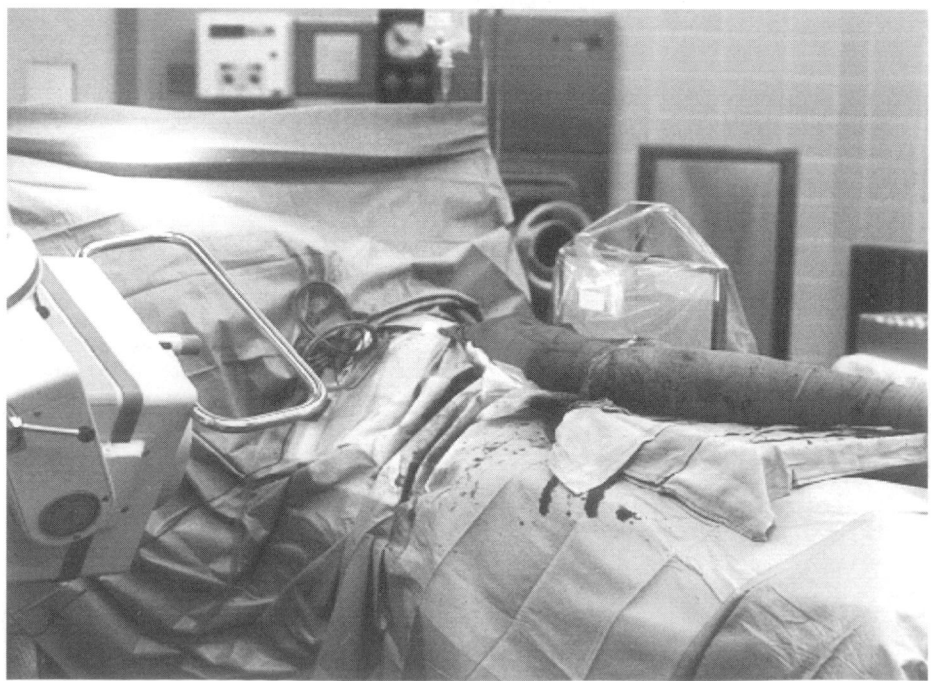

Figure 72.4 Correct positioning of the femur when shooting a cross-table view of the hip. Note how the knee is positioned upward with a stand to align with the axis of the body. This will promote a true ap or pa view of the hip.

73. INTRA-OPERATIVE KNEE
(AP VIEW)

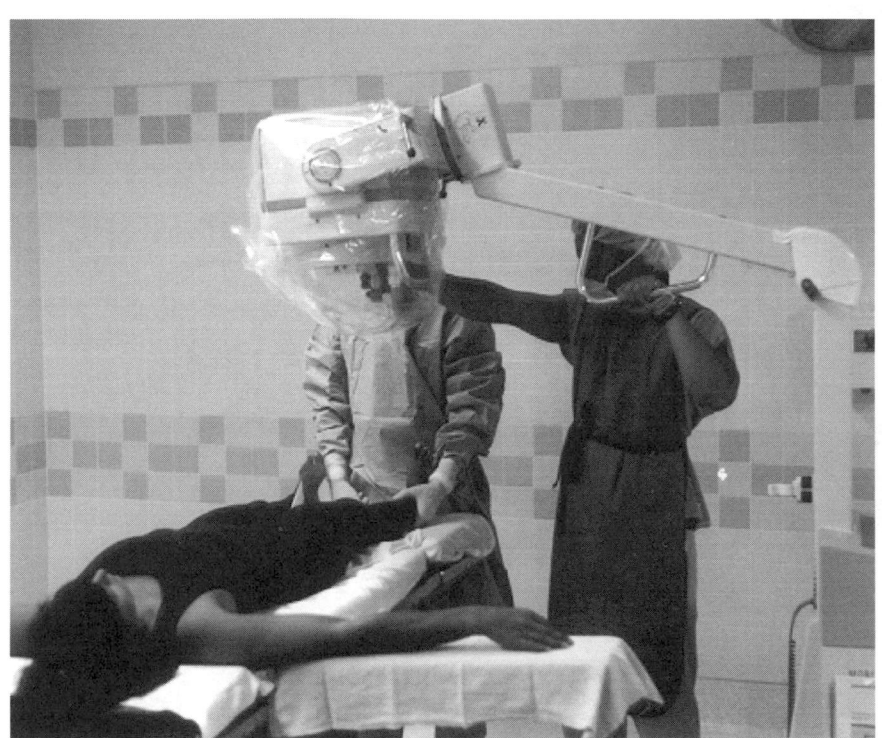

PATIENT POSITION: Patient will be supine.

X-RAY MACHINE: Portable X-ray will enter in the ap projection.

Notes: X-ray cassette will be covered with sterile drape.

Physician will place X-ray cassette on sterile field underneath patient's knee.

Cover portable tube with a sterile drape before positioning over knee.

Figure 73.1 *X-ray machine in position for ap view of the knee.*

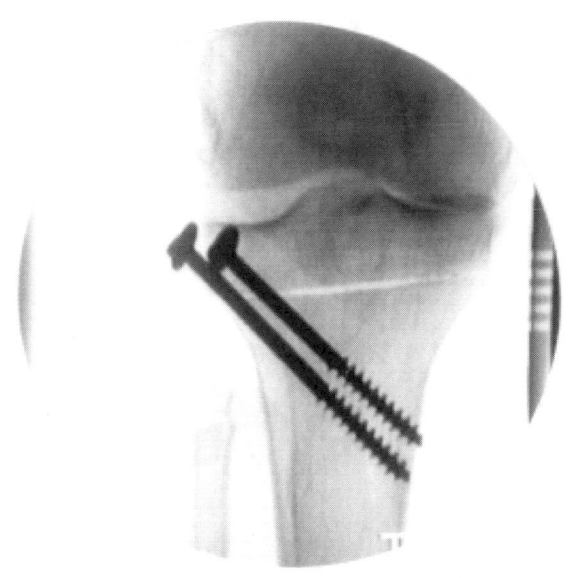

Figure 73.2 *X-ray image of ap knee with instrumentation.*

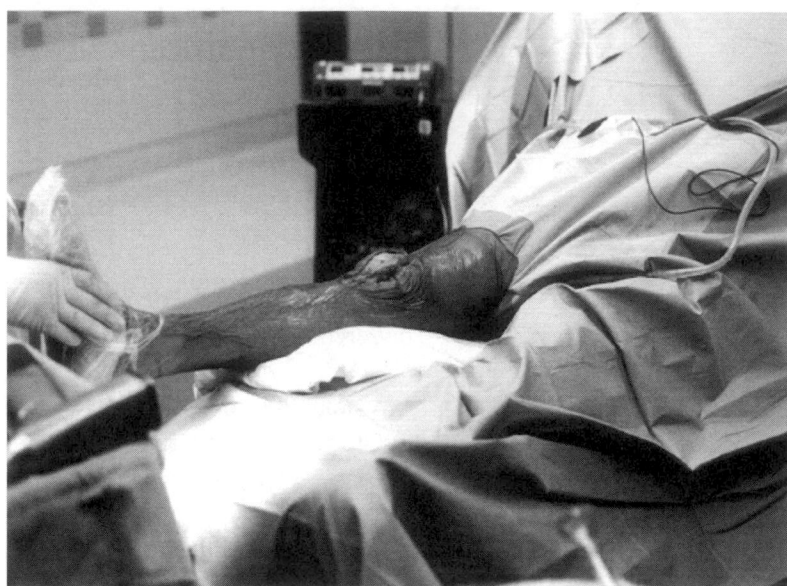

Figure 73.3 *Patient and cassette positioned for ap view of the knee. Foot is flexed to align the medial and lateral malleolus to obtain a true ap view of the knee.*

74. INTRA-OPERATIVE KNEE
(LATERAL VIEW)

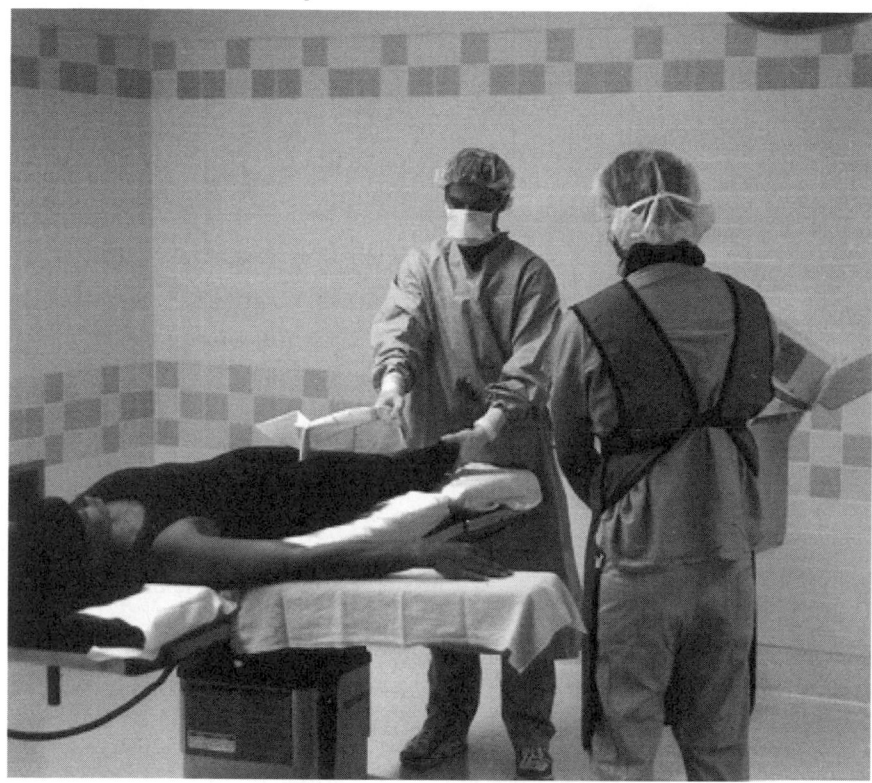

PATIENT POSITION: Patient will be supine with the knee extended.

X-RAY MACHINE: Portable X-ray will enter perpendicular to the patient with the beam parallel to the floor.

Notes: X-ray cassette will be covered with sterile drape.

Knee will have to be externally or internally rotated to create true lateral view.

The leg may have to be abducted or adducted to align the knee perpendicular to X-ray beam.

Figure 74.1 *X-ray machine and patient positioned for lateral view of the knee.*

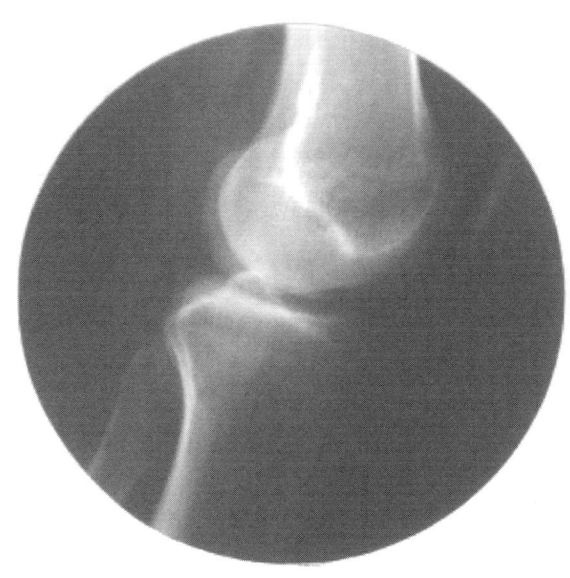

Figure 74.2 *X-ray image of lateral knee with instrumentation.*

75. INTRA-OPERATIVE ANKLE
(AP VIEW)

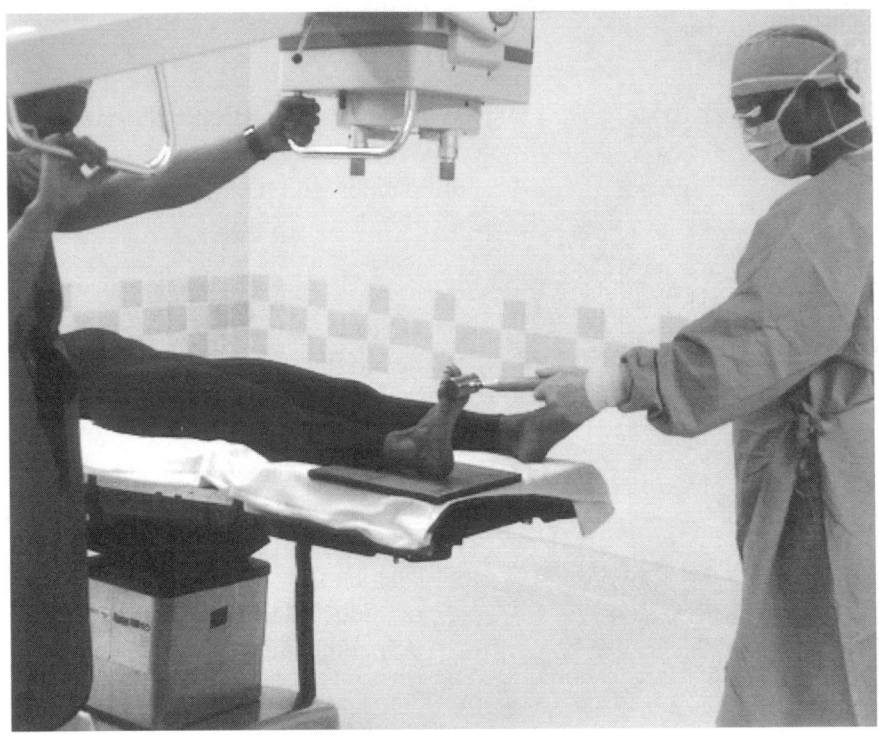

Figure 75.1 *X-ray machine in position for ap view of ankle.*

PATIENT POSITION: Patient will be supine. The affected ankle may be slightly raised with a bump.

X-RAY MACHINE: The portable X-ray machine will enter in the ap projection perpendicular to the patient.

Notes: Flex the foot to create a true ap view of the ankle.

Ensure that X-ray beam is perpendicular to the ankle.

Cassette must be covered with sterile drape before placing on sterile field.

Portable X-ray should be covered with sterile drape before placing over sterile field.

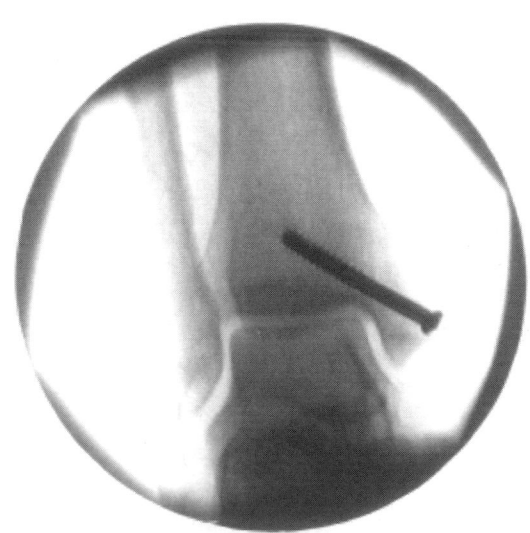

Figure 75.2 *X-ray image of ap ankle.*

INTRA-OPERATIVE ANKLE
(LATERAL VIEW)

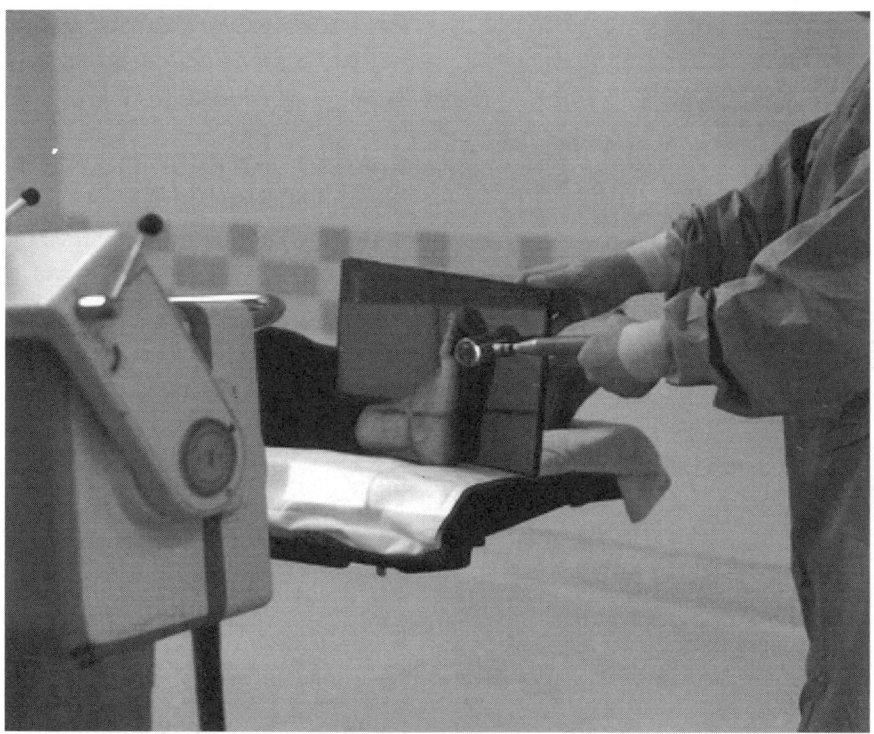

PATIENT POSITION: Patient will be supine. The affected ankle may be slightly raised with a bump.

X-RAY MACHINE: The portable x-ray machine will enter with the beam perpendicular to the ankle.

Notes: Flex the foot to create a true lateral of the ankle.

Ensure that beam is perpendicular and on line with the ankle.

Cassette must be covered with sterile drape when working in a sterile field.

Figure 76.1 *X-ray machine in position for lateral view of ankle.*

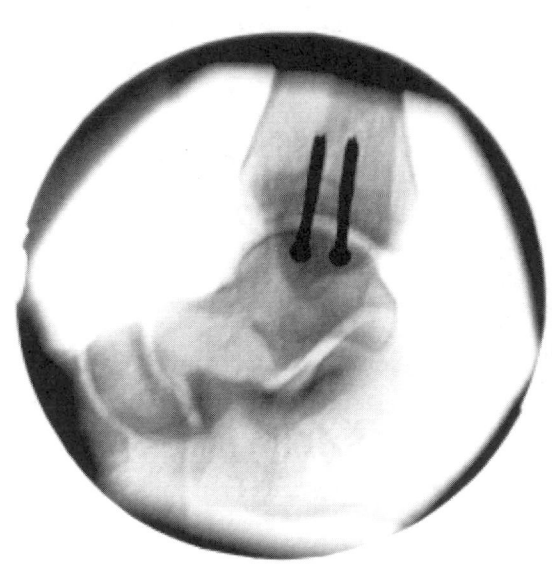

Figure 76.2 *X-ray image of lateral ankle.*

77. INTRA-OPERATIVE OS-CALCIS
(AP VIEW)

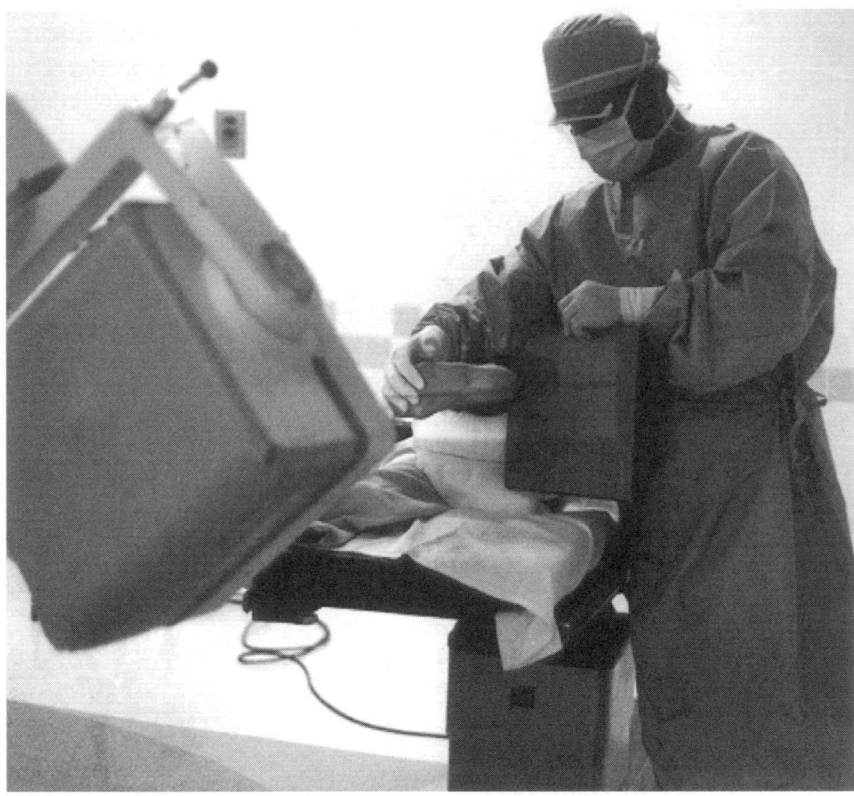

PATIENT POSITION: Patient will be in the lateral position with affected os-calcis up.

X-RAY MACHINE: Portable X-ray will enter at the patient's feet with beam pointed toward the head.

Notes: Cover cassette with sterile drape placed over the field.

Physician will flex the foot and place cassette posterior to os-calcis.

Angle the beam toward the head and centered on the mid foot.

Flexing the foot while in the lateral position and angling the beam toward the head is called the Mankey Technique.

Affected leg will be flexed at a 45-degree angle to the long axis of table.

Figure 77.1   X-ray machine and patient positioned for ap view of os-calcis (Mankey Technique).

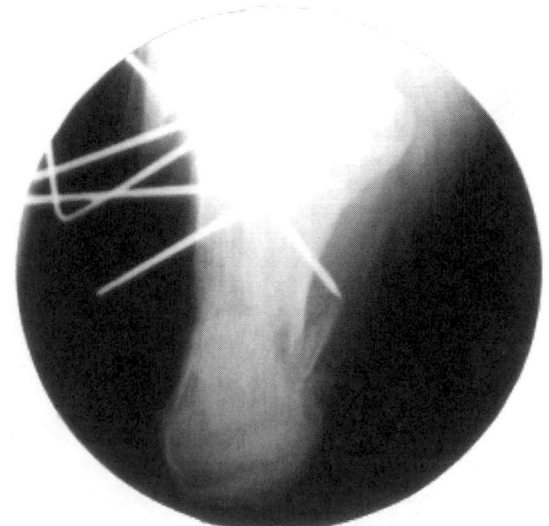

Figure 77.2   X-ray image of os-calcis with instrumentation.

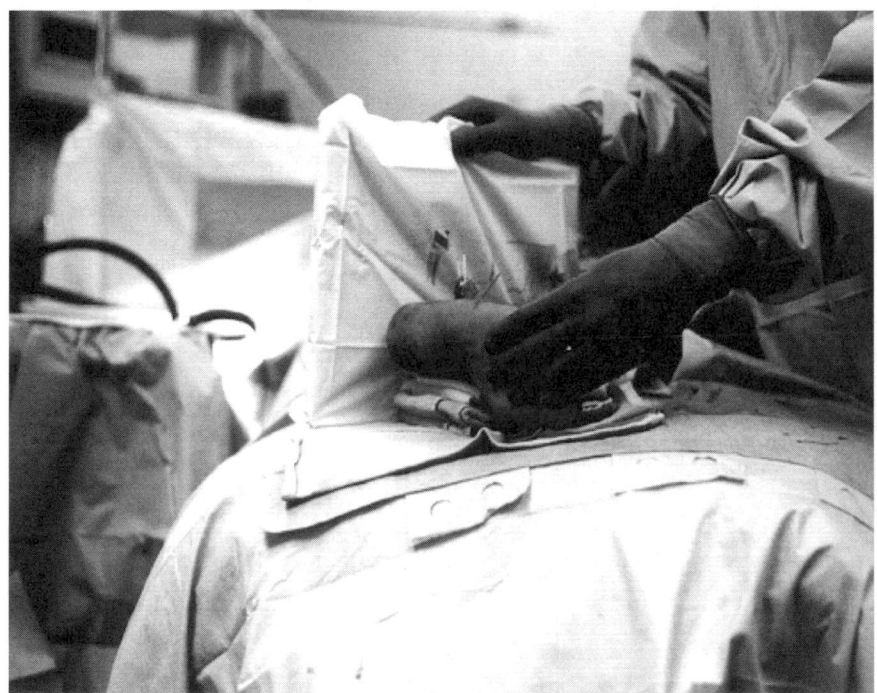

Figure 77.3 *When taking the intra-op os-calcis using the Mankey Technique, be careful of protruding pins so as not to puncture the sterile cover.*

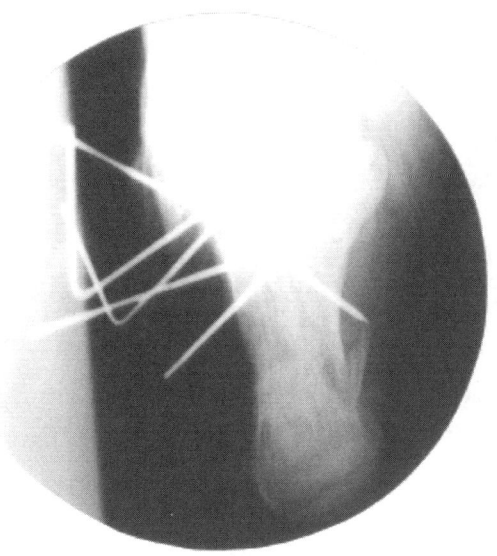

Figure 77.4 *X-ray image of os-calcis with pins protruding.*

78. INTRA-OPERATIVE OS-CALCIS
(LATERAL VIEW)

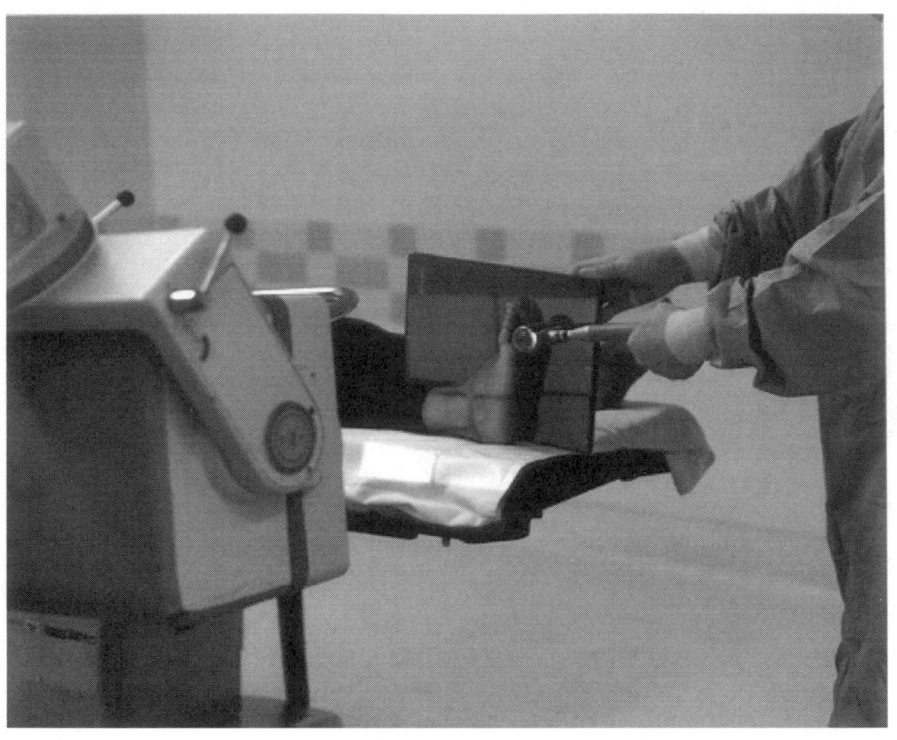

Figure 78.1 *X-ray machine and patient positioned for lateral view of os-calcis.*

PATIENT POSITION: Patient will be supine with affected foot up.

X-RAY MACHINE: Portable X-ray will enter lateral to the patient with the beam parallel to the floor.

Notes: X-ray tube will be covered with sterile drape placing over the field.

Table may have to be tilted to create a true lateral view.

Physician will place cassette with sterile cover medial to the effected os-calcis.

Angle X-ray tube if necessary to create a true lateral view.

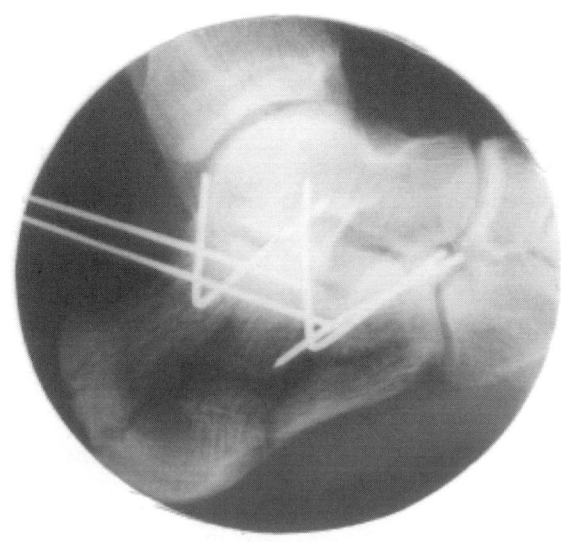

Figure 78.2 *X-ray image of lateral os-calcis.*

79. INTRA-OPERATIVE OS-CALCIS
(LATERAL VIEW, PATIENT IN LATERAL POSITION)

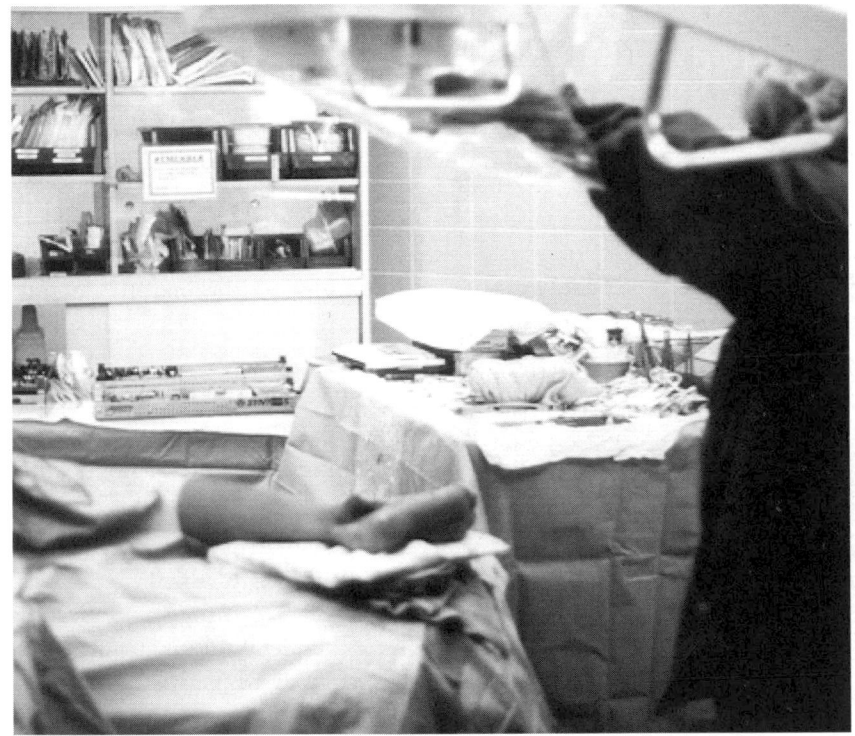

Figure 79.1 *X-ray machine in lateral projection of affected os-calcis.*

PATIENT POSITION: Patient will be in the lateral position with the ankle positioned to promote a true lateral view.

X-RAY MACHINE: Portable X-ray will enter in the lateral projection with the X-ray beam perpendicular to the floor and the cassette.

Notes: The ankle may have to be bumped up to obtain a true lateral view.

The portable X-ray will have to be covered with sterile cover when working over sterile field.

Surgeon will have to position cassette on sterile field. Cassette will be covered with sterile drape before placing over field.

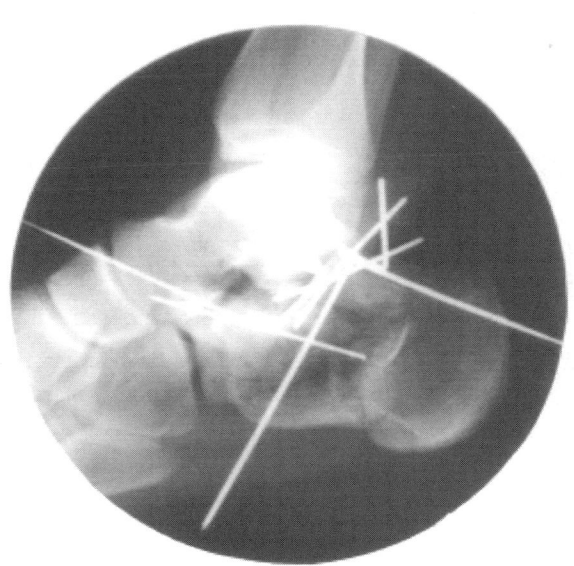

Figure 79.2 *X-ray image of os-calcis lateral view.*

80. INTRA-OPERATIVE LATERAL CERVICAL SPINE
(PRONE)

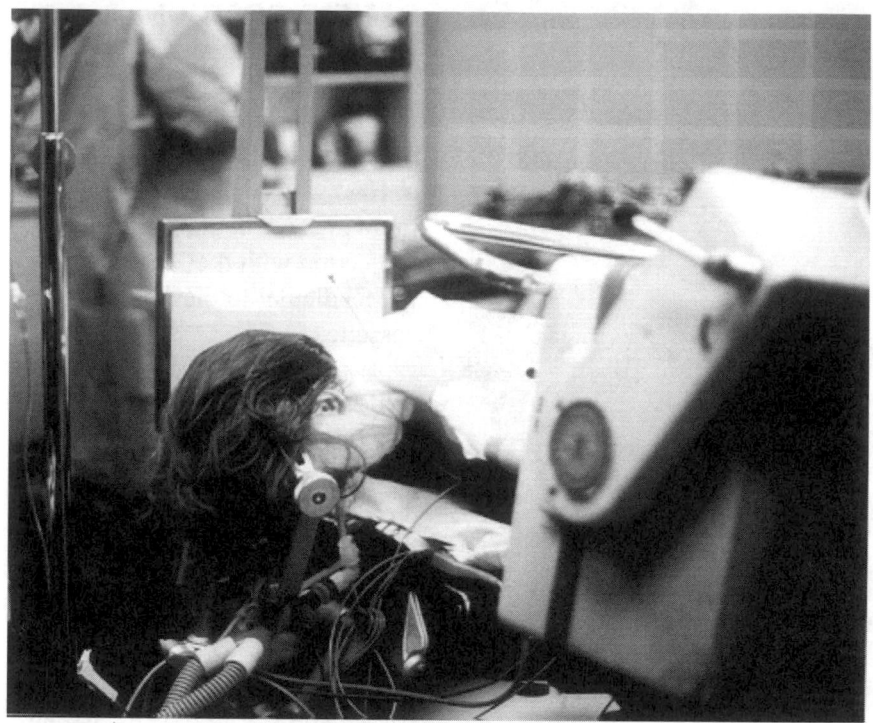

Figure 80.1 *X-ray machine positioned for lateral cervical spine.*

PATIENT POSITION: Patient will be either supine or prone depending on anterior or posterior approach.

X-RAY POSITION: Machine will enter perpendicular to patient and angled to obtain a true lateral view.

Notes: Align grid cassette along opposite side of the patient and perpendicular to the X-ray beam.

Ensure grid and beam are aligned to minimize grid cut-off.

X-ray beam should be centered to the grid and aligned with the spine.

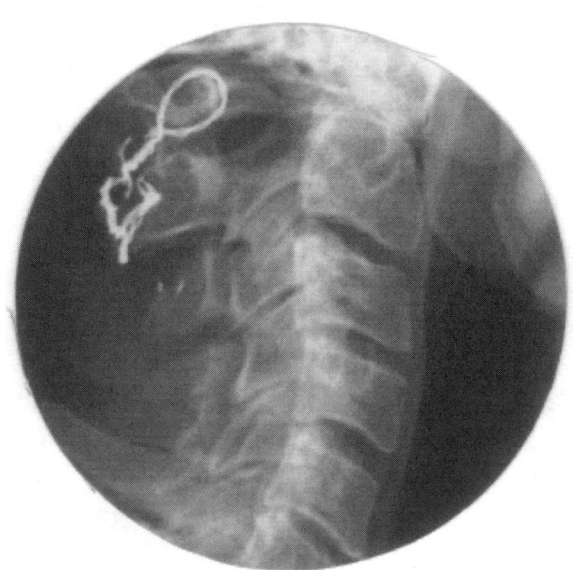

Figure 80.2 *X-ray image of lateral cervical spine with instrumentation.*

81. INTRA-OPERATIVE LATERAL CERVICAL SPINE
(SUPINE)

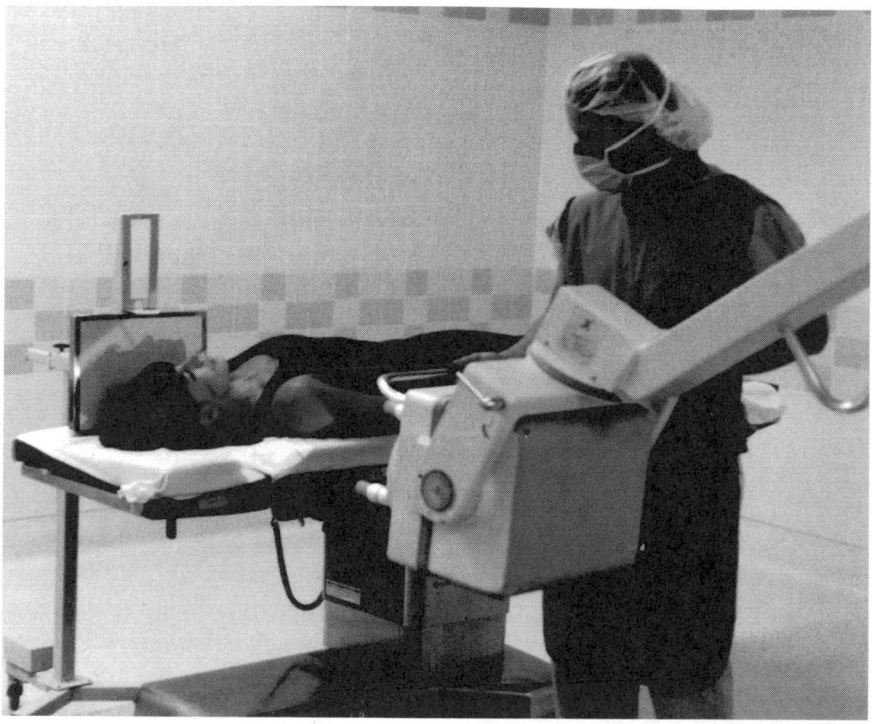

Figure 81.1 *X ray machine positioned for lateral cervical spine.*

PATIENT POSITION: Patient will be either supine or prone depending on anterior or posterior approach.

X-RAY POSITION: Machine will enter perpendicular to patient and angled to obtain a true lateral view.

Notes: Align grid cassette along opposite side of the patient and perpendicular to the x-ray beam.

Ensure grid and beam are aligned to minimize grid cut-off. X-ray beam should be centered to the grid and aligned with the spine.

Ensure the neck is rotated so the face is up to promote a true lateral.

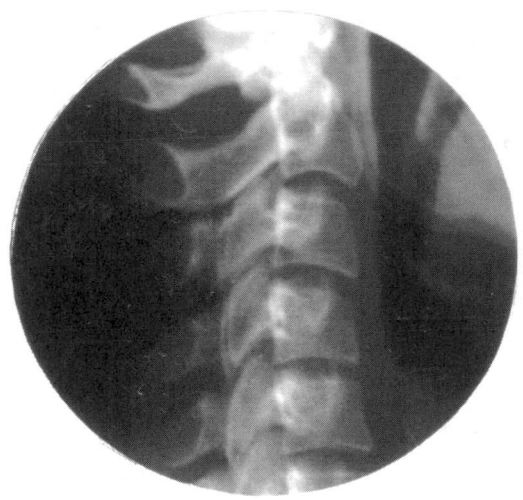

Figure 81.2 *X-ray image of lateral cervical spine with instrumentation.*

82. INTRA-OPERATIVE LATERAL CERVICAL SPINE

(PATIENT IN SITTING POSITION)

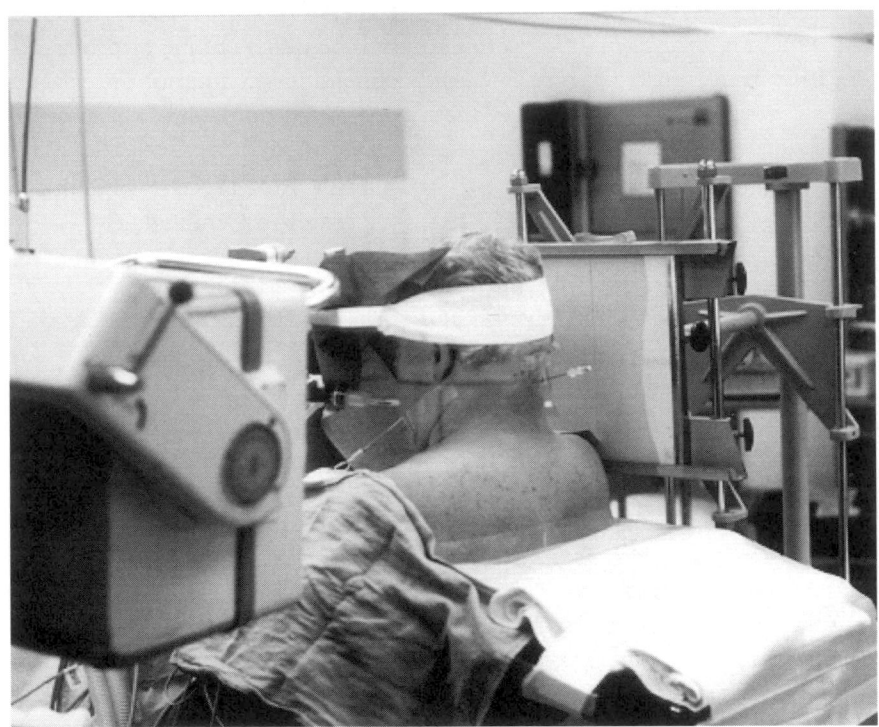

PATIENT POSITION: Patient will be in the sitting position with head held in harness.

X-RAY POSITION: Portable X-ray machine will enter lateral to the patient. The beam will be parallel to the floor and on line with the cervical spine.

Notes: Upright grid holder may have to be used for this exam.

Ensure X-ray beam is perpendicular to the grid cassette.

Use sterile cover to cover grid cassette when working on sterile field.

Figure 82.1 *X-ray machine positioned for lateral view of cervical spine.*

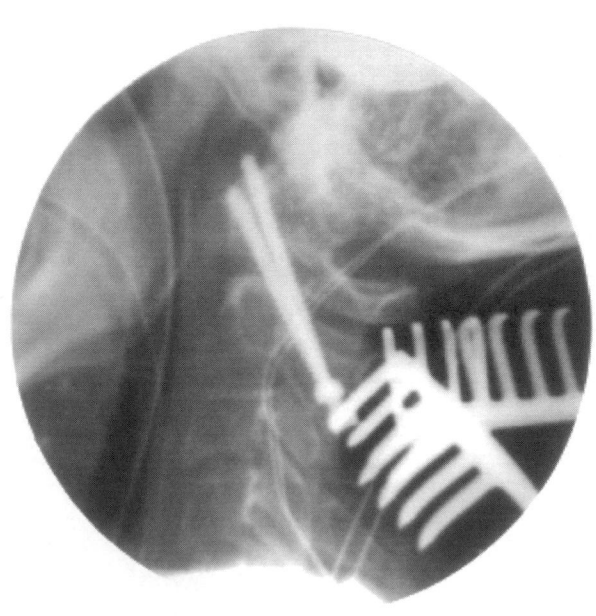

Figure 82.2 *X-ray image of lateral cervical spine.*

83. INTRA-OPERATIVE LUMBAR SPINE
(PA VIEW)

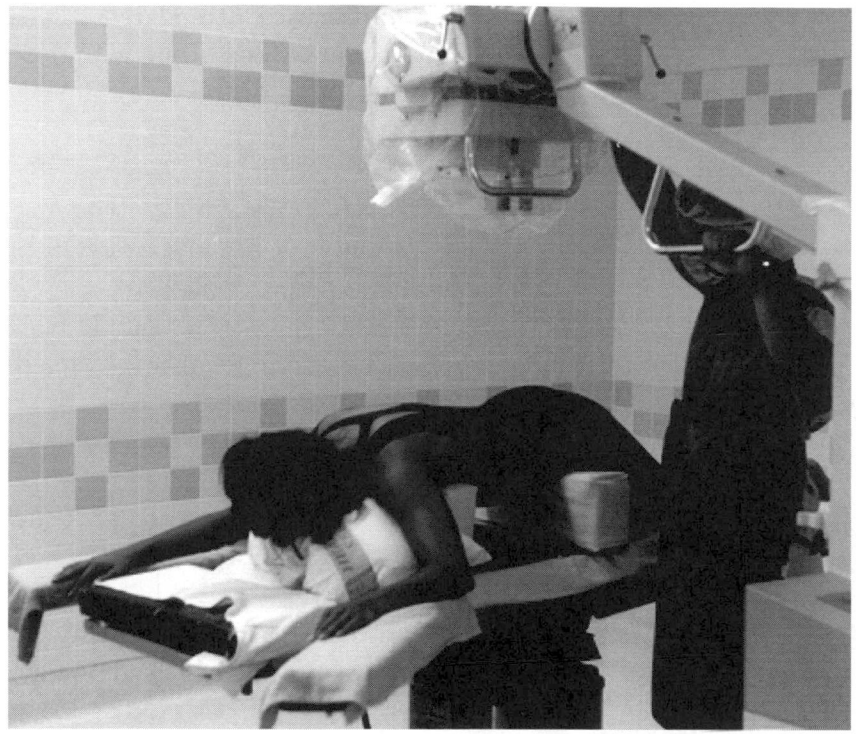

Figure 83.1 *X-ray machine in projection of pa spine.*

PATIENT POSITION: Patient will be prone with the spine area flexed on a frame device.

X-RAY MACHINE: The portable X-ray machine will enter perpendicular to the patient with the beam centered over the affected area.

Notes: Cover X-ray tube with sterile drape when working over a sterile field.

Ensure that beam is perpendicular to the grid cassette.

Pre-operative positioning is important to obtaining quality intra-operative views.

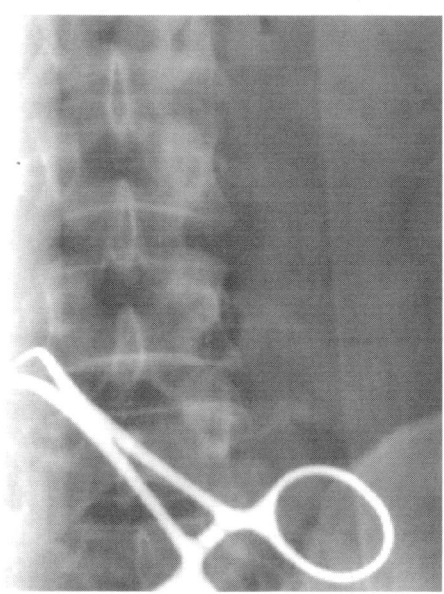

Figure 83.2 *X-ray image of pa spine.*

84. INTRA-OPERATIVE LUMBAR SPINE
(LATERAL VIEW)

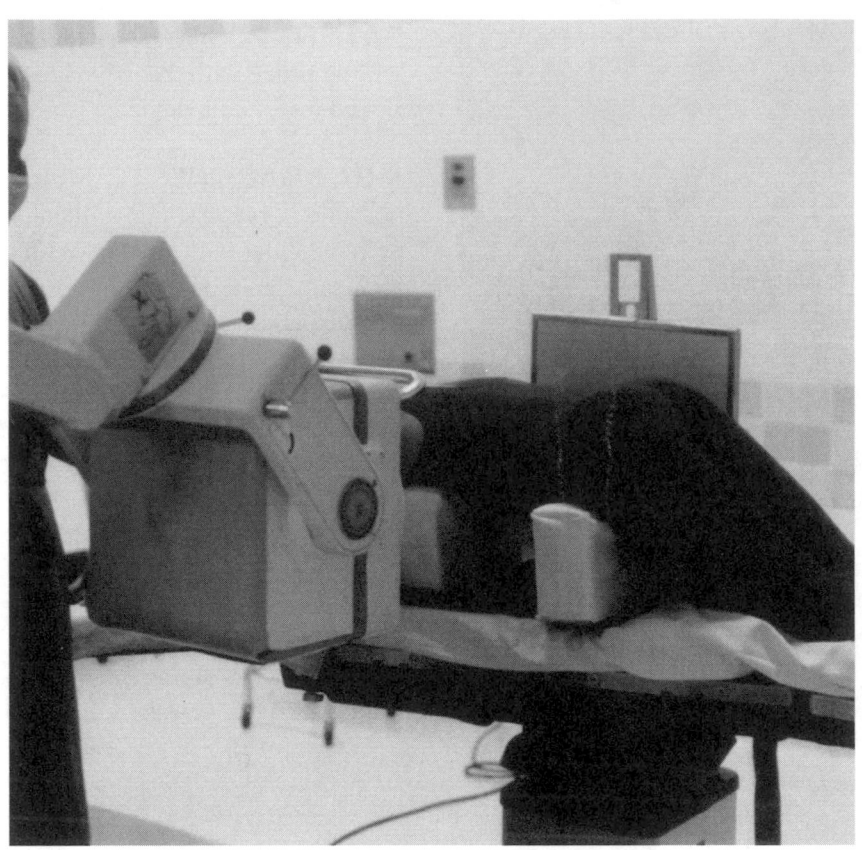

Figure 84.1 *X-ray machine in projection of lateral spine.*

PATIENT POSITION:
Patient will be prone with the spine area flexed on a frame device.

X-RAY MACHINE: The portable X-ray machine will enter perpendicular to the patient. The beam should be centered on the affected area in the lateral plane.

Notes: Ensure that grid cassette is perpendicular to the beam.

Grid cassette and the X-ray beam must be centered on the spine.

Ensure that X-ray beam is parallel to the floor.

Cover grid cassette with sterile cover when working over a sterile field.

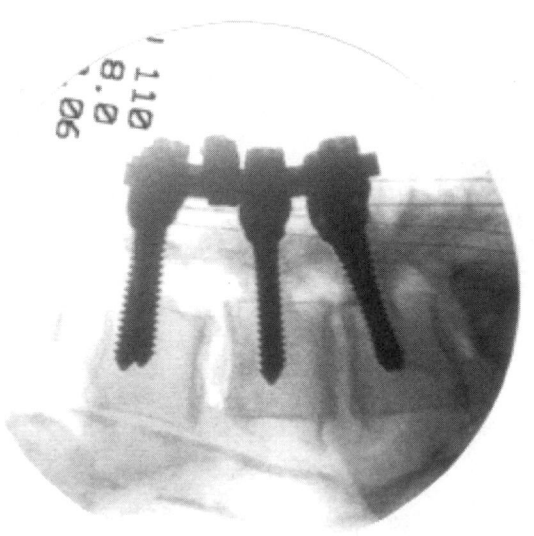

Figure 84.2 *X-ray image of lateral spine.*

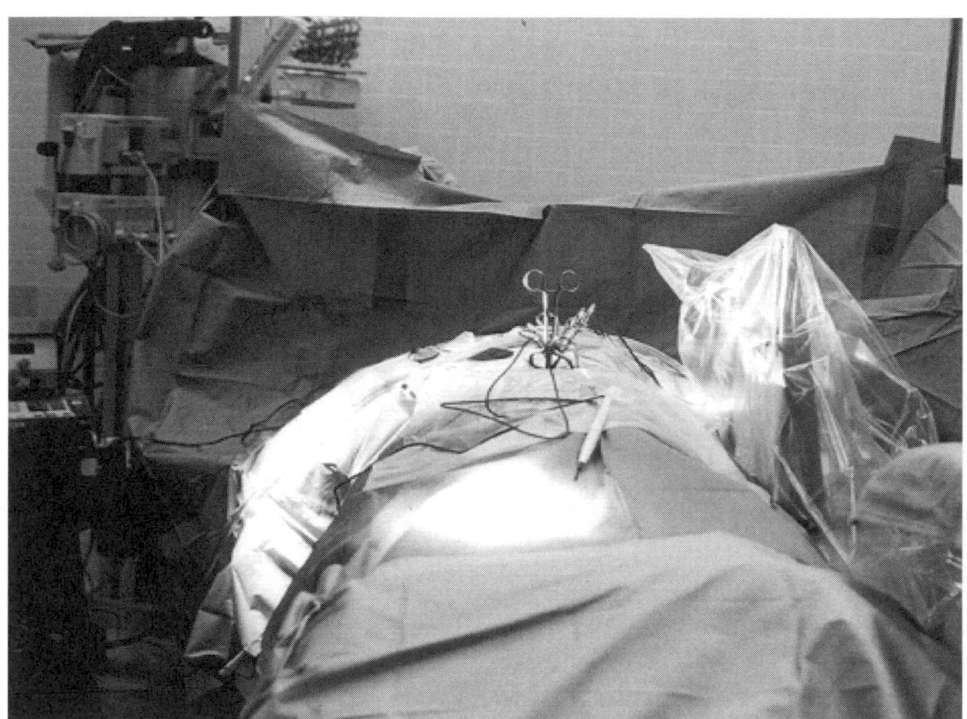

Figure 84.3 *When taking intra-operative films, remove all unnecessary instrumentation. This will reduce the scatter and promote a better-quality image.*

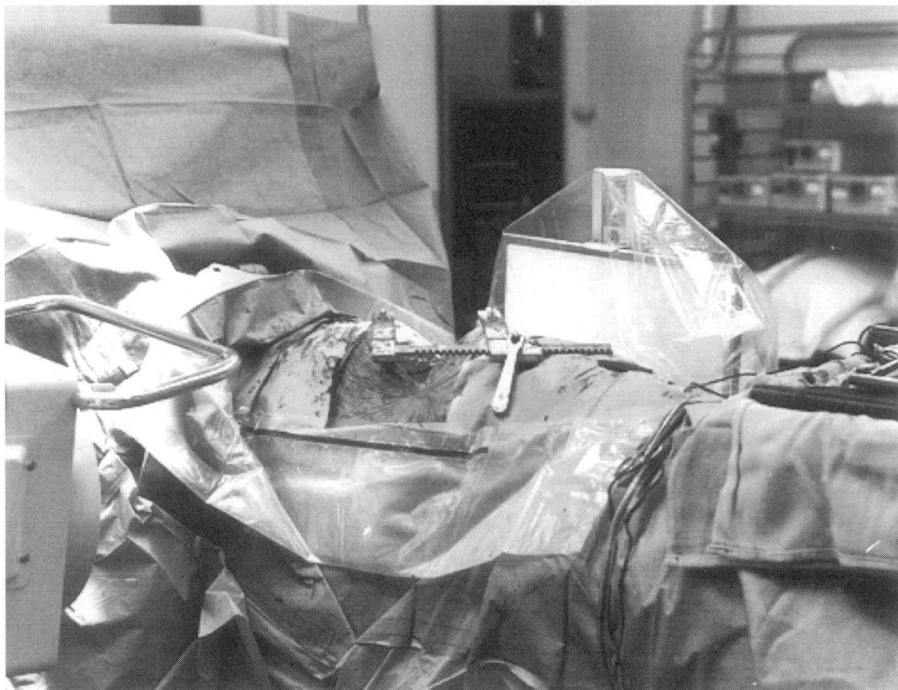

Figure 84.4 *Intra-operative cross-table ap spine being performed. All unnecessary instrumentation has been removed.*

85. INTRA-OPERATIVE T-SPINE
(AP VIEW)

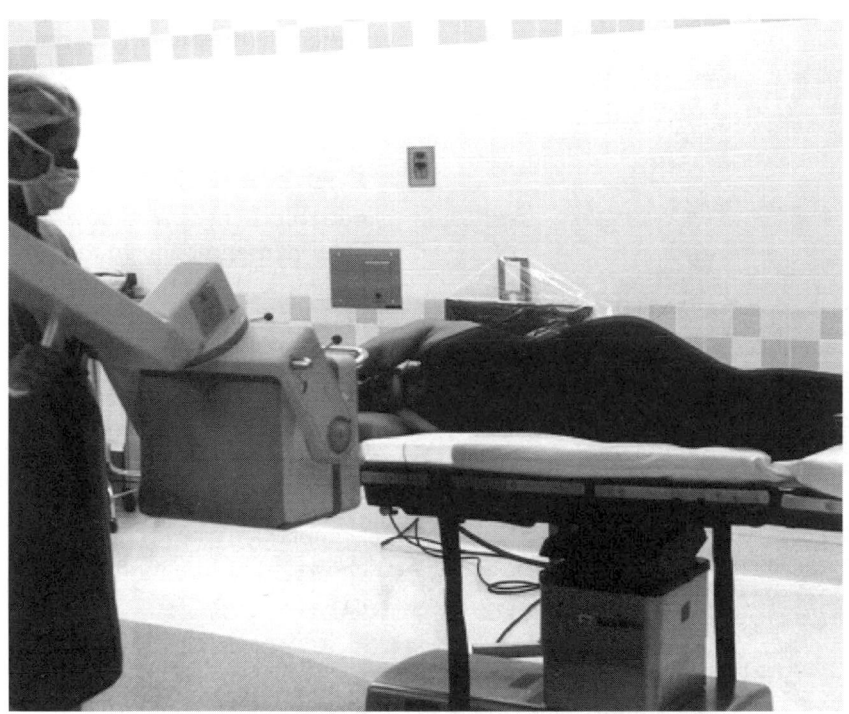

PATIENT POSITION: Patient will be in the lateral position with arms positioned above the shoulders.

X-RAY MACHINE: Portable X-ray will enter perpendicular to the patient with the beam parallel to floor.

Notes: Ensure that grid cassette is on line and perpendicular to the X-ray beam.

If working on sterile field cover grid cassette with sterile drape.

Figure 85.1 *X-ray machine and cassette positioned for cross table ap t-spine.*

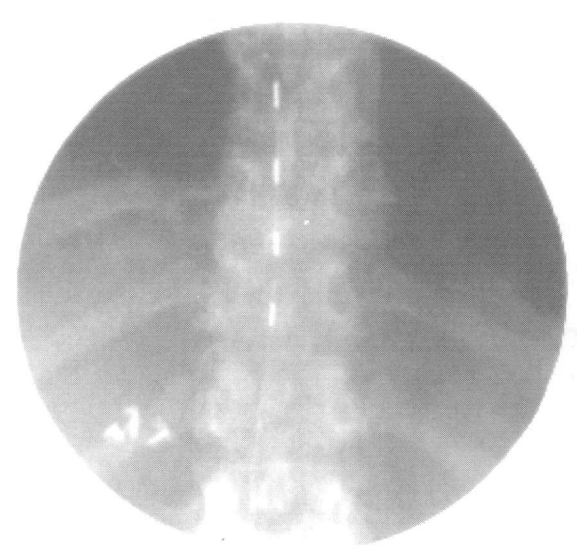

Figure 85.2 *X-ray image of ap t-spine.*

86. INTRA-OPERATIVE DECUBITUS CHEST
(AP VIEW)

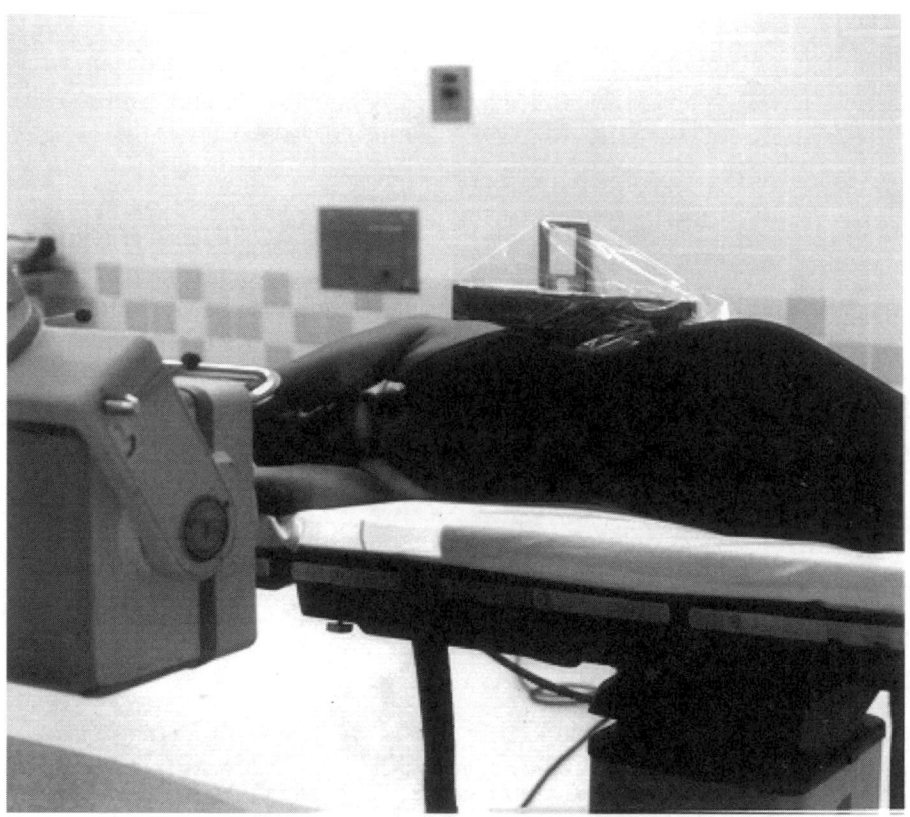

Figure 86.1 *X-ray machine and patient positioned for lateral Decubitus chest.*

PATIENT POSITION:
Patient will be lateral with the arms positioned above the head or forward of the turso.

X-RAY MACHINE: The portable X-ray machine will enter perpendicular to the patient with the beam parallel to the floor.

Notes: Cover cassette with sterile cover when working on sterile field.

Center X-ray beam on the chest and in line with the cassette.

Exposure should be made on inhalation of the chest.

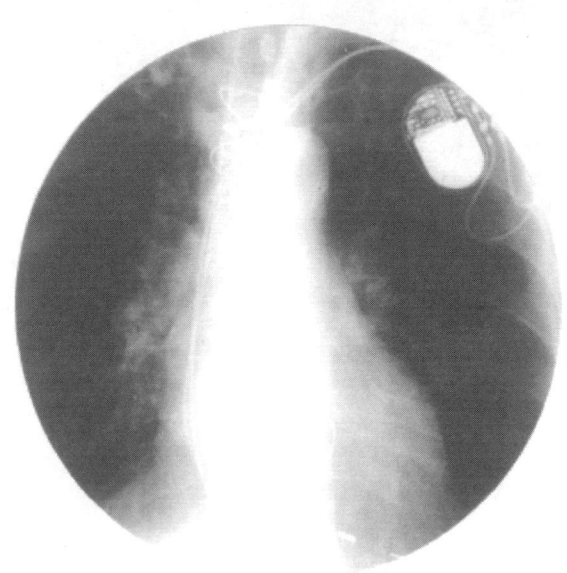

Figure 86.2 *X-ray image of Decubitus chest.*

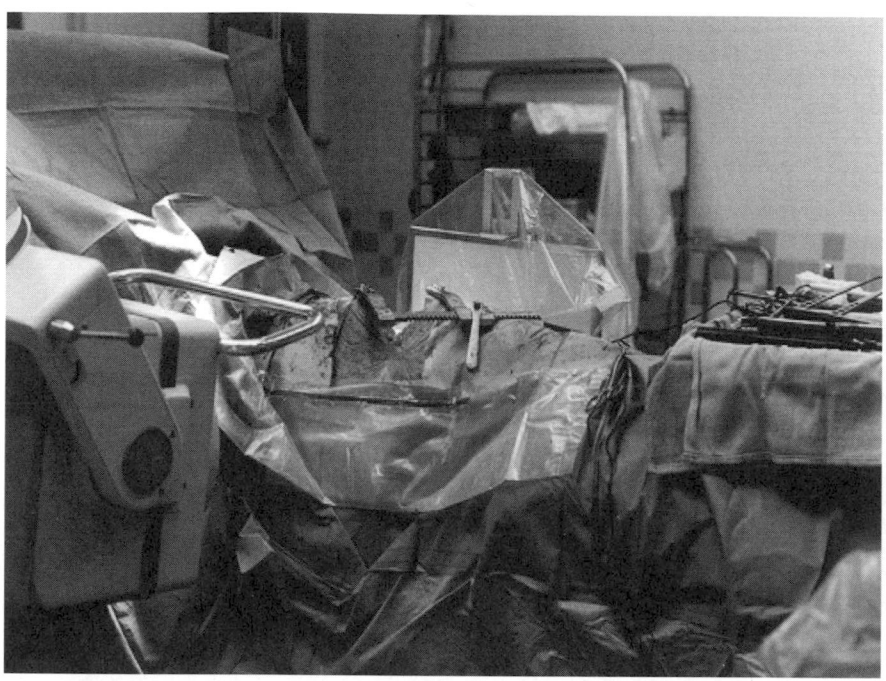

Figure 86.3 *A standard film holder covered with a sterile drape being utilized for a cross-table ap of the spine.*

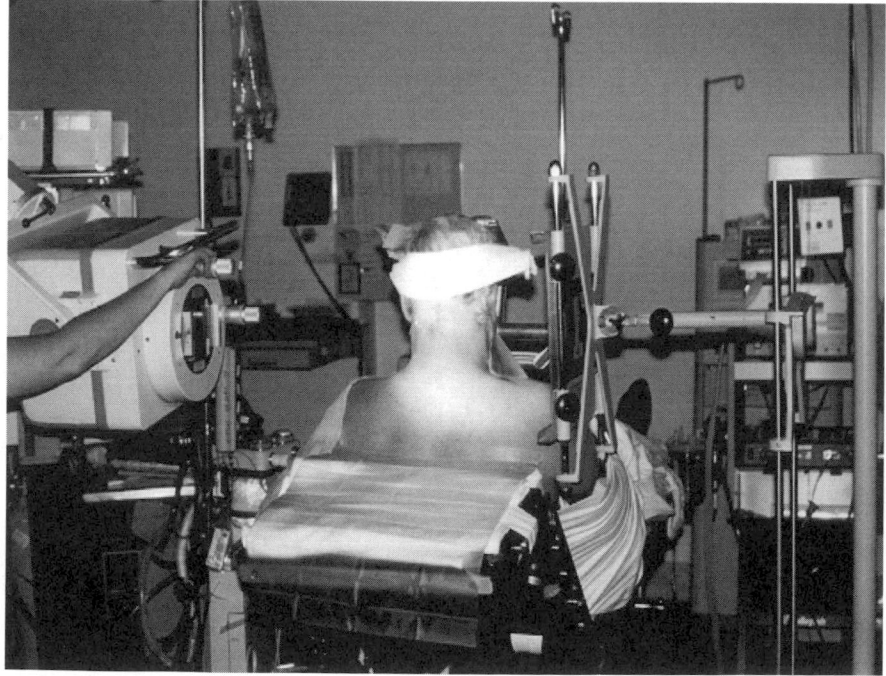

Figure 86.4 *An upright film holder being utilized for an upright lateral c-spine.*

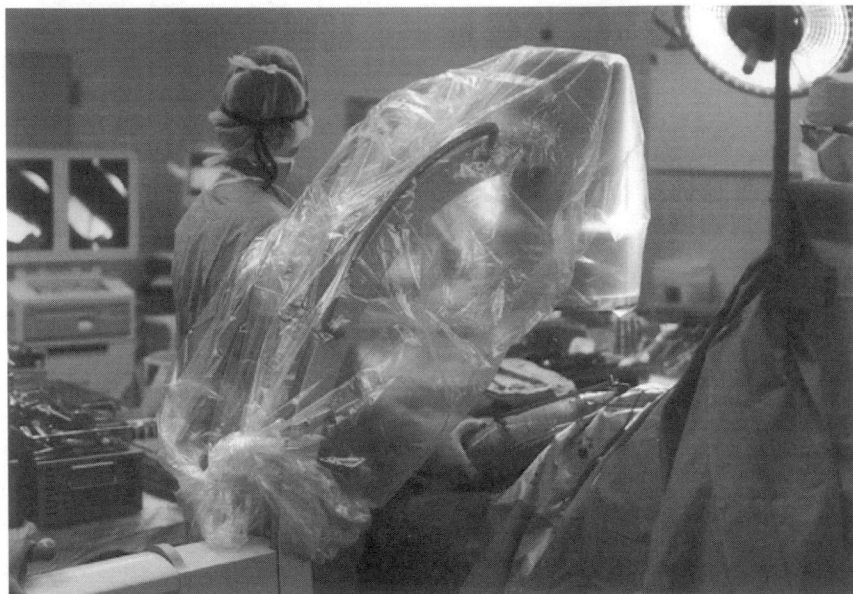

Figure 86.5 *The large c-arm drape being used. This type of drape should be used when close to sterile field.*

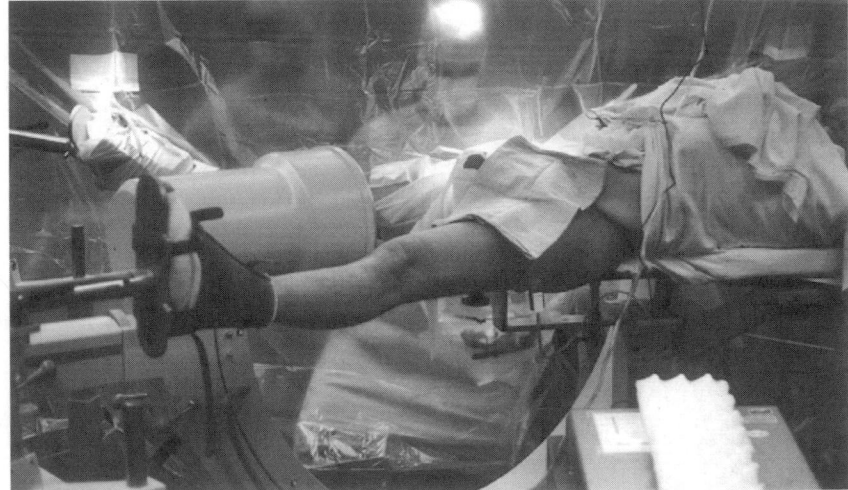

Figure 86.6 *The vertical isolation drape being used during a hip procedure.*

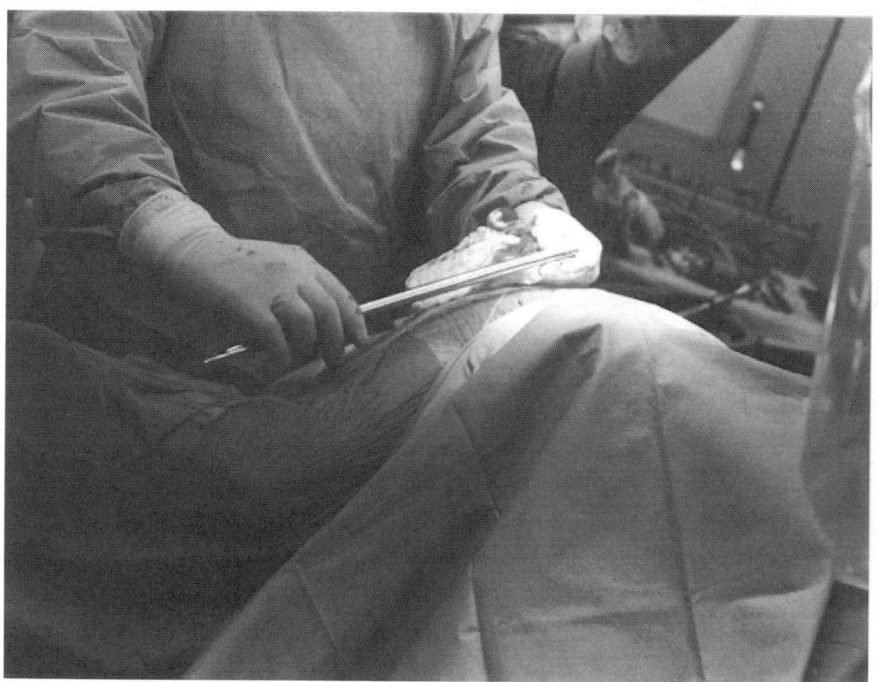

Figure 86.7 *Femur nail being measured to size of femur. When measuring nail length under fluoro, always show true views to ensure accurate length.*

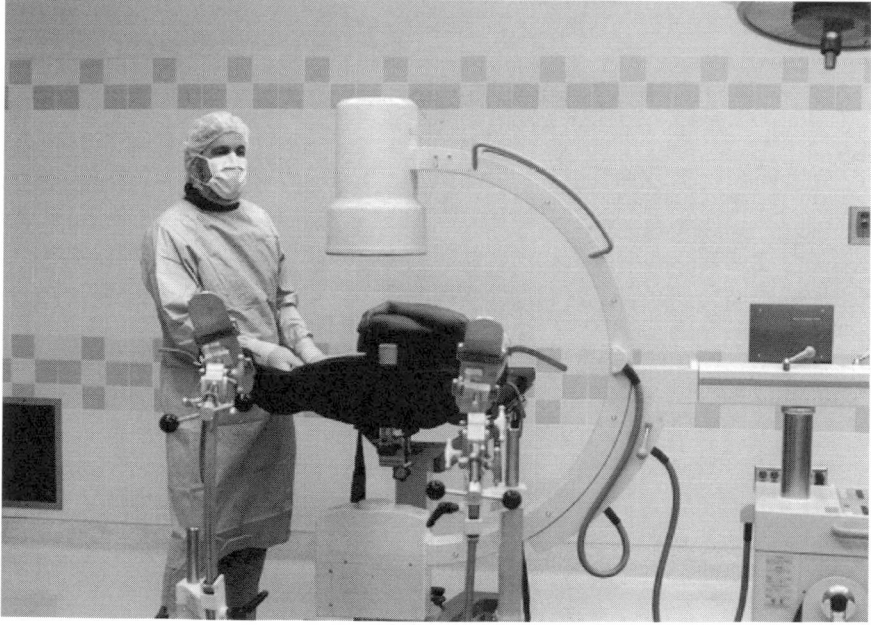

Figure 86.8 *Fracture table used during hip and femur repairs.*

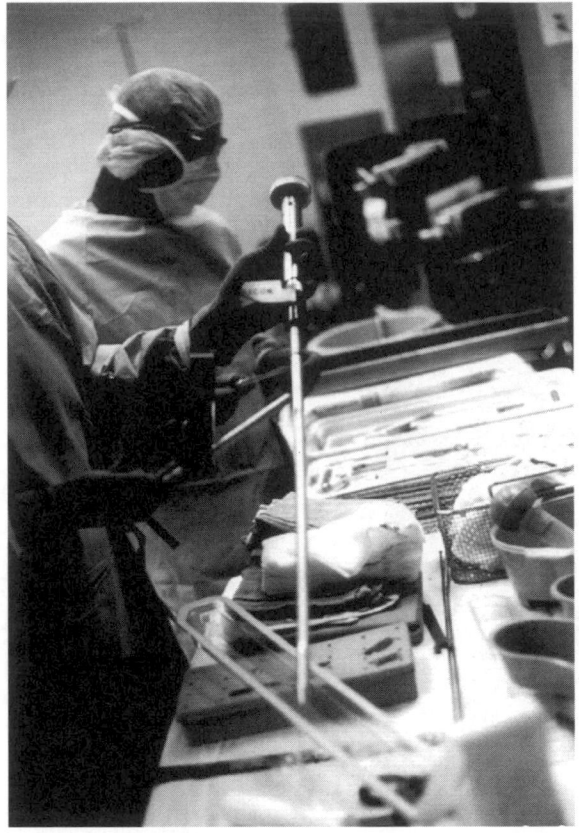

Figure 86.9 The femoral nail attached to the driving device ready for insertion.

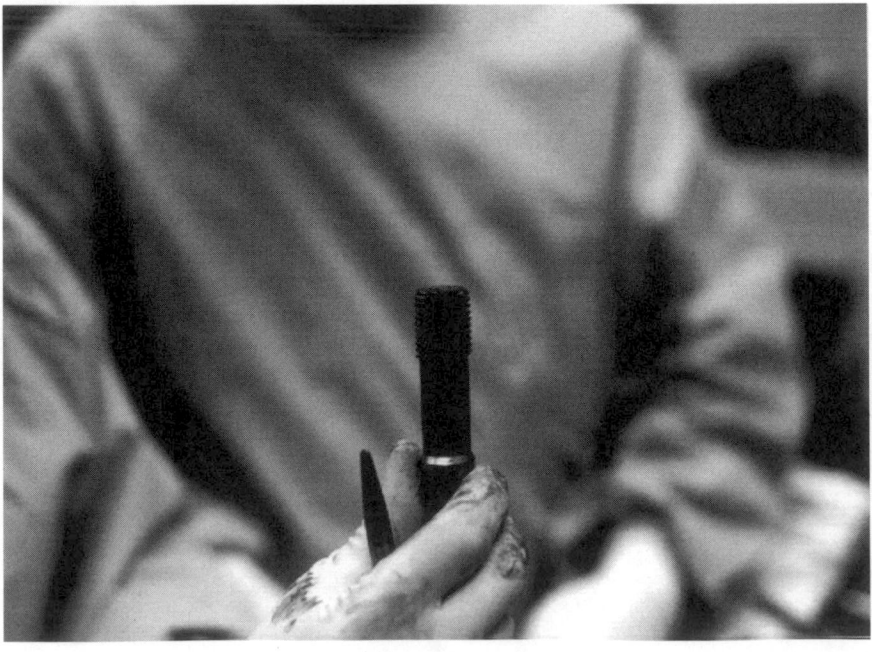

Figure 86.10 The cage spinal implant filled with bone graft before being inserted into the spine.

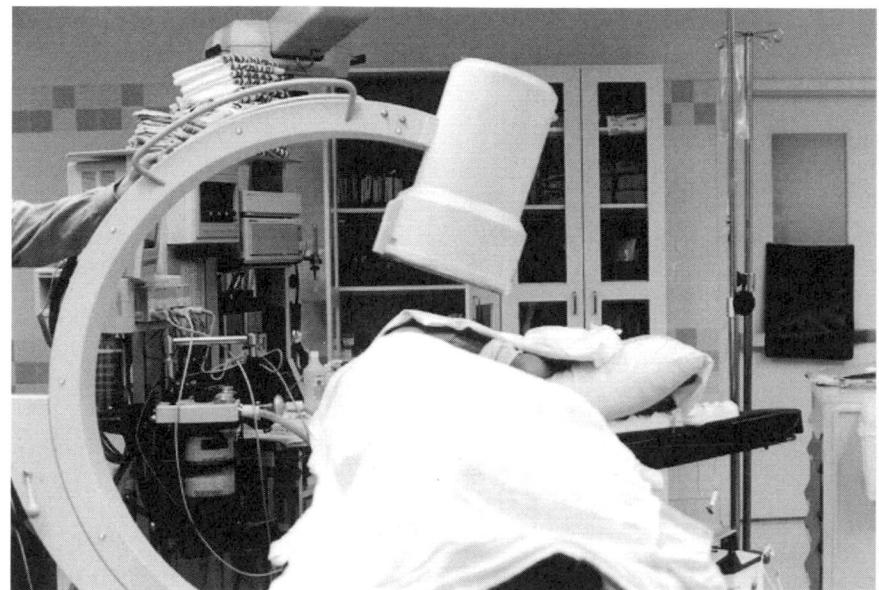

Figure 86.11 *The c-arm rotated in the moon-over position.*

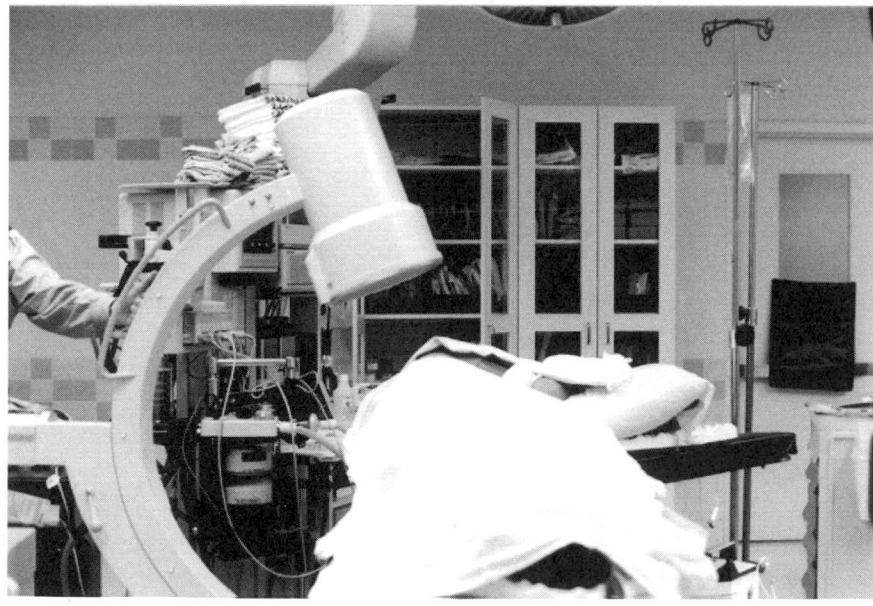

Figure 86.12 *The c-arm rotated in the moon-under position.*

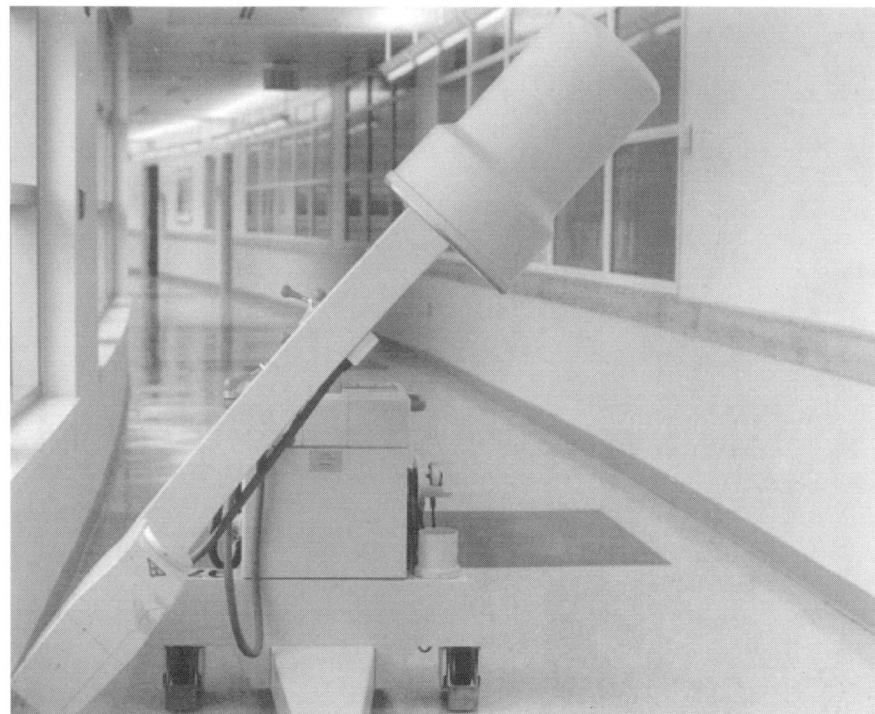

Figure 86.13 *The c-arm rotated in the sunrise position.*

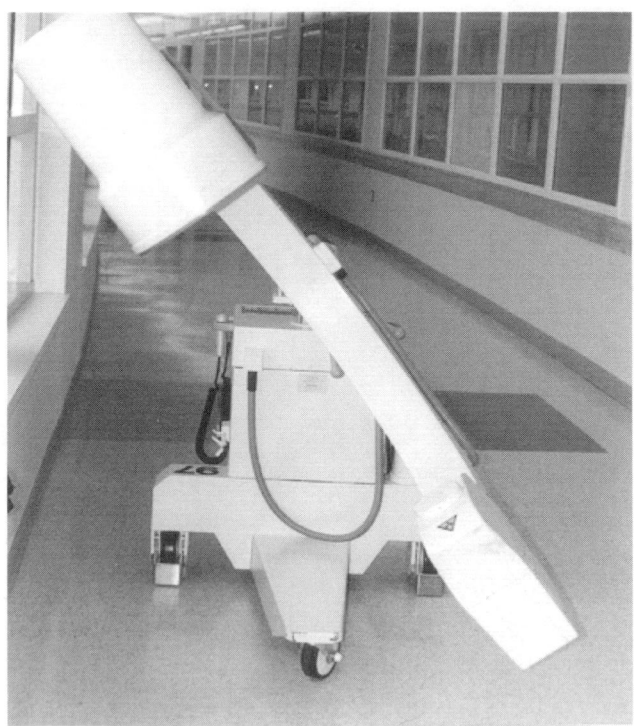

Figure 86.14 *The c-arm rotated in the sunset position.*

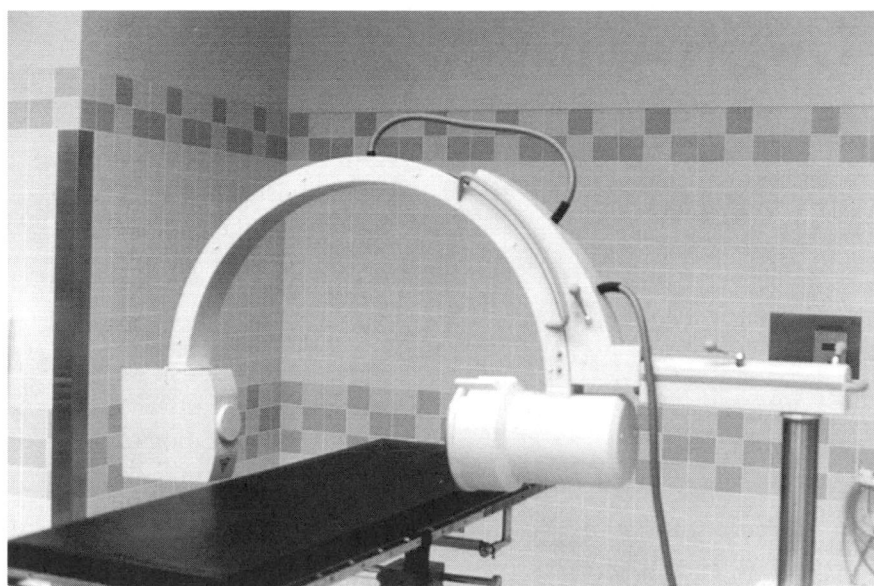

Figure 86.15 *The c-arm rotated in the over-the-top position.*

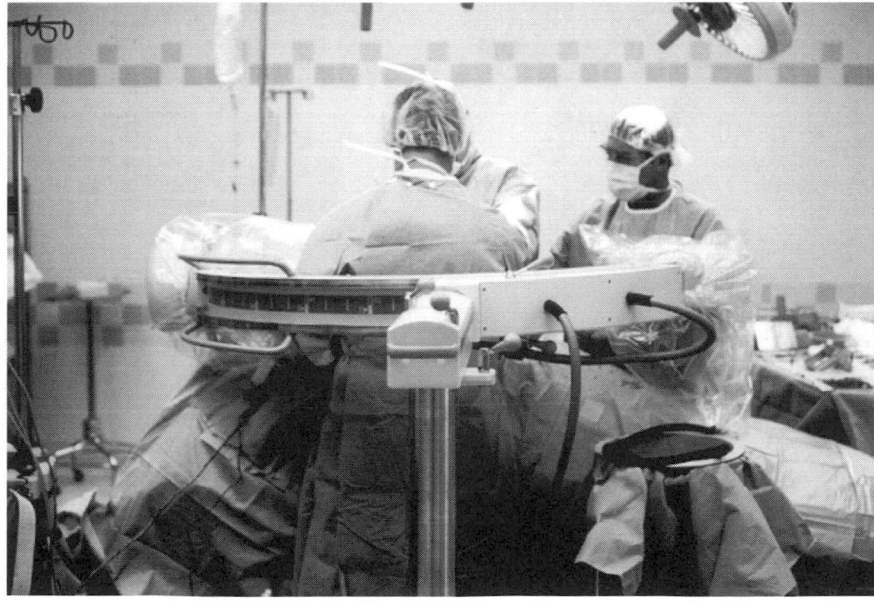

Figure 86.16 *The c-arm rotated in the horizon position.*

87(a). CORRECT POSITION OF TECHNOLOGIST FOR OPERATING C-ARM

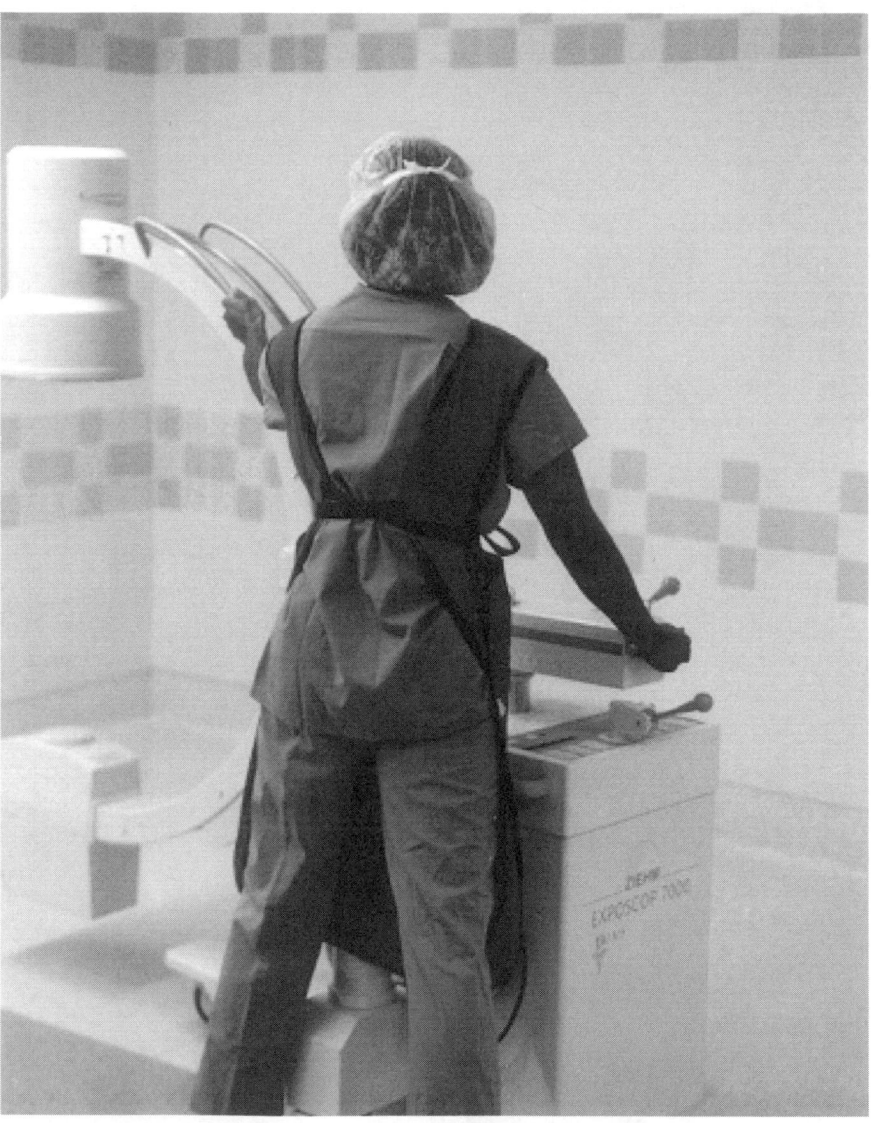

Technologist stands parallel to c-arm facing the control panel.

Allows for better viewing of the control panel.

Aids depth perception by allowing visualization of the anatomy in relation to the position of the image intensifier.

Allows the technologist to utilize body leverage, making manipulation of the c-arm easier.

Decreases the risk of lower-back injury to the technologist.

Figure 87(a) *Technologist standing in correct position for operating c-arm.*

87(b). INCORRECT POSITION OF TECHNOLOGIST FOR OPERATING C-ARM

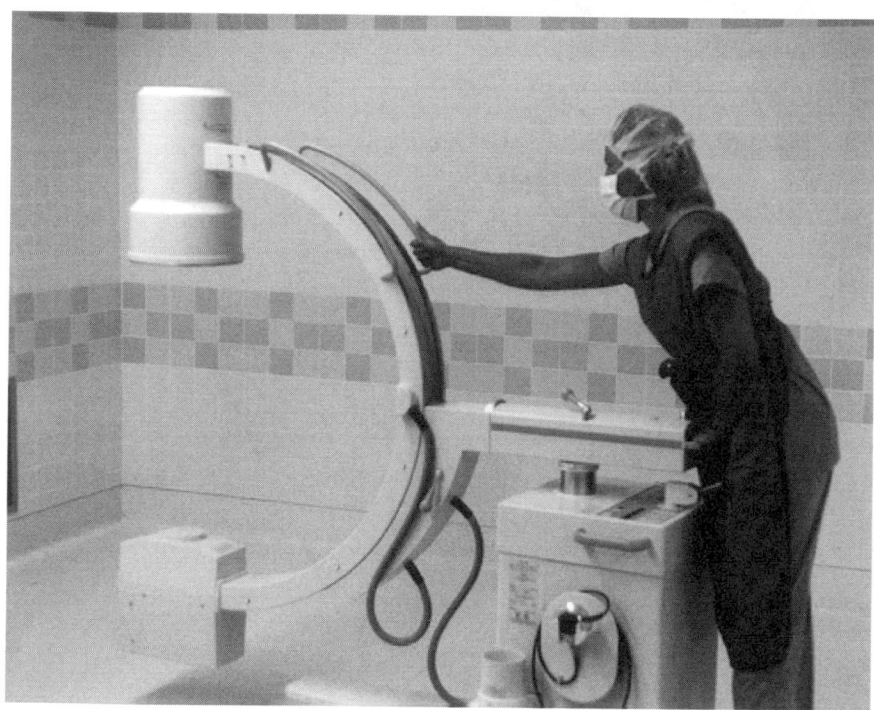

Technologist stands perpendicular to the control panel of the c-arm.

Angle limits the technologist's depth perception in viewing the relation between the anatomy and the position of the image intensifier.

Angle increases the risk of lower-back injury, as it causes the technologist to overextend and does not allow for the utilization of body leverage to manipulate the c-arm.

Figure 87(b) *Technologist standing in incorrect position for operating the c-arm.*

88. Handling of Cassette

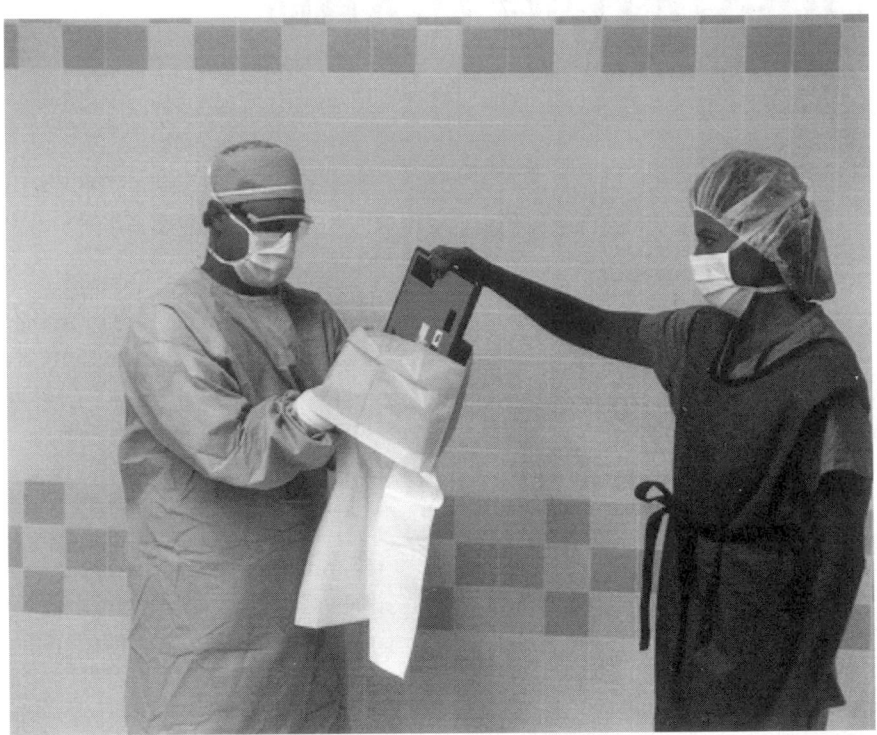

Figure 88.1 *When passing film onto sterile field for intra-op filming, gently place cassette inside cover keeping hands within the blue drape.*

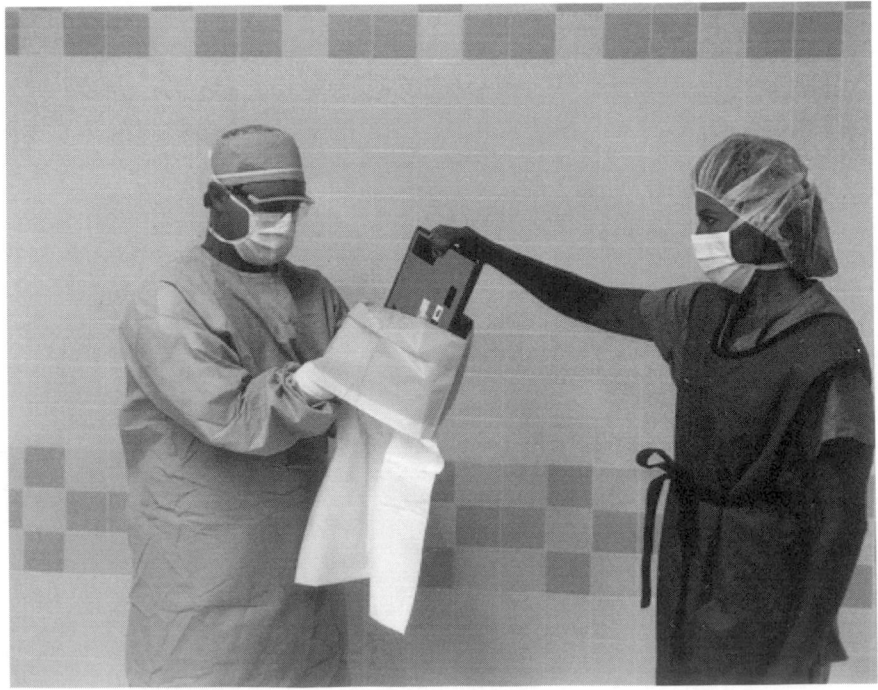

Figure 88.2 *Once cassette is placed inside cover, gently pull off blue cover, keeping hands inside the drape area.*

Appendix

Abducted	Drawn away from the median plane or from the axial line of a limb
Adducted	Drawn toward the median plane or toward the axial line of a limb
AP	Anterior to posterior
Auld	Instrument used to make a starting point
Bump	To place an object to assist with positioning of anatomy
Cannulated	To introduce a cannula, which may be left in place
Caudal	Directed toward the feet
Cephalad	Directed toward the head
Decompression	Relief of pressure by means of surgery
Fluoro	Continuous fluoro from the c-arm
Image intensifier	Camera portion of the c-arm that processes the X-ray image
Inlet view	Position to view the superior aperture of the minor pelvis, bonded by the crest and pecten of the pubic bones
Internal fixation	Fixation that is placed inside or within
Interbody	Occurring within the medullary canal
LAO	Left anterior oblique
Laparoscopy	Using instrumentation for examination of the interior
LPO	Left anterior oblique
Osteotomy	Removal of a wedge of bone
Outlet view	Position to view the lower aperture of the pelvis inferior
PA	Posterior to anterior
PCL	Posterior cruciate ligament
Prone	Lying face downward
Proximal	Closer to any point of reference, as opposed to distal
Pulse fluoro	Intermittent fluoro
Radiopaque	Not penetrable by roentgen rays or other forms of radiant energy
Radiolucent	Permitting the passage of roentgen rays or other forms of radiant energy
Reverse Trendelenberg	Having the feet tilted down from the supine position
ROA	Right anterior oblique
RPO	Right posterior oblique
Snap cover drape	Banded drape covering image intensifier and allowing mobility of c-arm
Snapshot fluoro	One-shot program on the c-arm that restricts the image to one picture
Supracondylar	Situated above a condyle or condyles
Supine	Lying on the back with the face upward
Telescope	To move the c-arm in and out without moving the base
Trendelenberg	Head tilted downward from the supine position
Valgus	Bent outward, twisted, denoting a deformity in which the angulation of the part is away from the midline of the body
Varus	Bent inward, denoting a deformity in which the angulation of the part is toward the midline of the body
Vertical isolation drape	Hanging drape that isolates an entire sterile area
Wig-wag	The lock that allows side-to-side movement of the c-arm without moving the base

Surgical Procedures

Alcohol celiac plexus block	Nerve block of the spine using alcohol. Patient is usually prone.
Back cage	Spinal fusion device used between the body of the spine with bone graft and metal cage
Cannulated screws	Screws placed within the femoral head for fracture fixation
Decompression hip screw (DHS)	Fixing of a fractured hip with screws and slide plate
Epidural catheter	catheter placed within the dural space of the spine
Femoral nailing	Rod placed inside the femoral cortex for fixation of a fracture
Fletcher suit implant	Examination using fluoroscopic guide to insert radioactive implant into the cervix area
Greenfield filter placement	Filter placed within the artery to collect blood clots and promote flow
Hip arthroscopy	Arthroscope of the hip using the c-arm to check distraction of the femur and location of the scope in the hip
Hip osteotomy	Osteotomy of the hip with screw or plate fixation
Hip revision	Replacement of an existing total hip. C-arm is used to insure removal of cement and to check prosthesis position
Humeral nailing	Rod placed inside the humeral cortex for fixation of a fracture
Laparoscopic Cholangiogram	Removal of the gall bladder through the scope with contrast injected to highlight the ducts
Omaya Reservoir	Port placed within the skull using fluoroscopic guide to relieve cranial pressure
Pacemaker/AICD insertion	Electronic pacing device placed within the heart ot assist with cardiac stability
PCL Repair	Repair of the posterior crusciate ligament in the knee with c-arm assistance
Percutaneous ultrasonic lithrotripsy (PUL)	Used to break up large stones within the kidney
Radioactive seed implant	Procedure using fluoroscopic guide to insert radioactive seeds into the prostate
Radioactive frequency rhizotomy	Frequency probes are placed within the rhizotomy nerves to stimulate the facial area
Shunt placement	Tube catheter placed within the skull to relieve cranial pressure
Steffee plating	Fusion of the lumbar spine using pedicle screws and plates
Supracondylar femoral nail	Retrograde femoral nail placed with the starting point at the knee for distal femur fractures
Tibial nailing	Rod placed inside the tibial cortex for fixation of a fracture
Transphenoidal resection of pituitary tumor	Resection of pituitary tumor assisted with the c-arm to confirm location

Surgical Views

Anderson's View	View obtained during a cervical-one spinal fusion with the c-arm angled caudal to view of body of cervical one
Crutcher's View	View obtained when doing hip arthroscopy with the patient supine. Rotate the c-arm over the top 5 to 10 degrees while tilting the c-arm 10 to 15 degrees cephalad.
Dupen's View	View of the lumbar spine when patient is prone. Obtain by wig-wagging the c-arm to open the disc space.
Flugstad's View	View of the AP shoulder during total shoulder procedures, obtained by angling the c-arm 5 to 10 degrees caudal while rotating over the top 5 to 15 degrees
King's Technique	Intentional angling of the x-ray beam and the grid cassette to align with a patient's scoliosis during anterior/posterior spinal fusion procedures
Laurnen's View	View obtained with the c-arm by using an angle to align with the stenosis
Mankey's Technique	Taking an intra-operative os-calcis with the patient lateral
Raisis' View	View obtained with the c-arm lateral by rotating the c-arm to superimpose the orbit and center the pituitary
Toomey's View	View of the AP hip with the c-arm angled 5 to 7 degrees cephalad while rotating over the top 8 to 15 degrees
Winquist's View	View of the femur during femoral nailing. Rotate the c-arm over the top 10 to 15 degrees while tilting toward the head of the femur 5 to 10 degrees.

C-Arm Positioning Terminology

Horizon	Tilting the c-arm so that the image intensifier and the tube are parallel to the surface
Moon over	Rotating the c-arm over the top of the patient without moving the base
Moon under	Rotating the c-arm back under the patient without moving the base
Pan	Scanning the c-arm up or down the patient's body while moving the base
Sunrise	Tilting the c-arm to the left without moving the base
Sunset	Tilting the c-arm to the right without moving the base
Top over	Tilting and rotating the c-arm to view the ap or p.a. view from the top. This is used when the table does not allow for underneath movement.
Wag	Moving the c-arm to the right without moving the base
Wig	Moving the c-arm to the left without moving the base